Additional Praise for

Healing PCOS

"There's so much health information swirling around out there, it's hard to know where to begin. And then you meet Amy Medling and everything begins to make sense. This book is *the* guide to living and thriving with PCOS. It's powerful, practical, and delivered with equal parts tough love, bear hugs, and hope."

—Jessica Murnane, author of *One Part Plant* and
   founder of Know Your Endo

"For many, a polycystic ovary syndrome diagnosis can be scary and isolating. Amy Medling shares her inspiring journey of challenges and triumph with PCOS, infertility, and other symptoms. *Healing PCOS* offers much-needed comfort and hope for those struggling with PCOS, and a 21-day lifestyle plan with valuable resources for transforming into PCOS Divas."

—Sasha Ottey, MHA

"A diagnosis like PCOS tends to come with a lot of rules, prohibitions, and a sense of limitation that can feel both daunting and oppressive. Amy Medling's book provides an empowering perspective that can make all the difference. Her book shows you the path of truly living and thriving. *Healing PCOS* outlines the steps that can lead you from a black-and-white prescription to a technicolor, vibrant life."

—Melissa McCreery, PhD, author of *The Emotional Eating
   Rescue Plan for Smart, Busy Women*

"*Healing PCOS* is a must read for any woman diagnosed with this disorder who is struggling to regain power over her health. Writing from her personal journey of trial and error, Amy provides a step-by-step guide for women to find their own path to health and, ultimately, joy in life. With a 21-day plan covering diet, exercise, and mindfulness, Amy provides women with the essential knowledge and tools needed to live their best lives."

—Jennifer Koslo, PhD, RDN, CSSD, LD, CPT, author of *The Insulin
   Resistance Diet for PCOS* and *The Complete DASH Diet for Beginners*

"PCOS exacts a physical and emotional toll on women. Though many of my patients find the lack of a cure particularly devastating, Amy Medling's approach, outlined in an easily digestible, action-oriented fashion in *Healing PCOS*, helps restore a sense of control and establish a series of goals that would honestly help every one of us be healthier and happier! Women struggling with their PCOS diagnosis should turn to this resource for an uplifting how-to on achieving their wellness goals."

—Rashmi Kudesia, MD, MSc, reproductive endocrinology
and infertility specialist

"*Healing PCOS* is a helpful guide that contains everything a woman needs to know to understand and conquer her PCOS. In only 21 days, readers will learn how to heal themselves from the inside out by adopting a healthy diet, moving naturally, meditating, and repeating positive affirmations. I wish I had access to a detailed yet easy-to-read book such as this when I was first diagnosed with PCOS!"

—Tara Spencer, author of *PCOS Diet for the Newly Diagnosed*

"*Healing PCOS* is a timely, practical, and well-tested plan for creating sensible and lasting health changes for women with PCOS. The plan is laid out in an easy-to-utilize fashion that makes sense, and Amy's recommendations are all gentle, sound, and appealing. Her plan offers strategic and comprehensive support for living a physically, mentally, and spiritually balanced life with PCOS."

—Dr. Gretchen Kubacky, "The PCOS Psychologist"
and founder of PCOS Wellness

"*Healing PCOS* by Amy Medling is a generous, accessible, and practical invitation and road map for those with PCOS to create a personalized healing plan that allows them to thrive. With gentle encouragement, well-researched methods, and specific but not strident guidance, *Healing PCOS* inspires your inner diva and guides you into discovering what *you* most need to heal from the inside out. With wholehearted warmth and a time-tested approach, Amy compassionately empowers you to take control of your health so that you can more naturally feel the way you most want to feel and profoundly restore your hope."

—Rosie Molinary, author of *Beautiful You: A Daily Guide
to Radical Self-Acceptance*

healing
PCOS

AMY MEDLING

healing
PCOS

A 21-DAY PLAN

for Reclaiming Your Health and Life
with Polycystic Ovary Syndrome

HarperOne
An Imprint of HarperCollinsPublishers

HarperOne

FIRST HARPERCOLLINS PAPERBACK EDITION PUBLISHED IN 2019

Designed by SBI Book Arts, LLC

Library of Congress Cataloging-in-Publication Data is available upon request.

ISBN 978-0-06-274817-1

19 20 21 22 23 LSC 10 9 8 7 6 5 4 3 2 1

Contents

Foreword

I met health coach and PCOS Diva Amy Medling online when she invited me to speak on a PCOS Diva podcast. I had heard wonderful things about her from my patients with polycystic ovary syndrome (PCOS), who praised Amy's inspiring website and coaching. I was delighted to finally meet Amy in person in Atlanta at the 2016 PCOS Challenge Conference. Amy is a serene and peaceful woman who radiates love and intelligence.

According to the Androgen Excess and PCOS Society, PCOS affects 5 to 15 percent of women worldwide. PCOS is associated with multiple symptoms ranging from irregularly spaced menstrual periods to hair loss, weight gain, and elevated blood pressure. In spite of the wide array of symptoms, PCOS is commonly regarded as a reproductive disorder, and most women with it are prescribed the birth control pill. However, no birth control pill can prevent metabolic problems or the development of type 2 diabetes. Furthermore, the role of a healthy lifestyle cannot be underestimated. American medicine is not equipped to provide the support for a healthy lifestyle in the broadest sense with regard to nutrition, movement, and spiritual health.

Derived from her own experience, Amy's approach to PCOS stems from a health-based point of view rather than the disease-based paradigm of conventional medicine. Where conventional medical treatment is designed to pursue the enemy with a well-aimed bullet, Amy coaches about the fundamentals of self-care and the importance of eating well, moving regularly, and maintaining a positive mindset. This is not to say that medication can't help PCOS, but without self-care the effect of medication is minimal.

Healing PCOS is an informative and inspiring step-by-step guide to learning to cherish yourself. Before you jump into changes in diet and exercise, Amy asks you to be mindful, create goals, and change the way you talk to yourself. With love and acceptance, she reminds readers that powerful women are not victims.

—Katherine D. Sherif, MD
Director, Jefferson Women's Primary Care;
Professor and Vice Chair, Department of
Medicine, Thomas Jefferson University

Foreword

Amy Medling and I share the same mission: to help women with PCOS optimize their health and take control of their lives. If you are among them, we want you to feel strong, vibrant, joyful, and self-assured so that you can achieve your personal goals. I'm confident that reading *Healing PCOS* and following the plan Amy outlines in it will help set you on a path to health and healing.

Like Amy, I also have PCOS and had to travel my own path of self-discovery to find my way to health and joy. I experienced many of the same letdowns she did and had to self-diagnose, despite seeing "world-class" doctors at a major university medical school. Now we both take an integrative and holistic approach to the treatment of PCOS.

As a physician, board certified in both OB/GYN and Integrative Medicine, with a special expertise in PCOS, I order an array of tests to evaluate my patient's inflammation, immune, and nutrient status; food allergies and sensitivities; gut microbiome; epigenetics; heavy metals and toxic load; and hormonal levels. But all the fancy tests in the world will have no real value for you if you do not address stress control, adequate and quality sleep, proper nutrition, and regular movement and fitness. In addition, embracing the concepts of living in the moment and having self-love is absolutely crucial for optimal health. The advice contained in *Healing PCOS* is the very foundation of care for women with PCOS, offering you the tools to take control of your health, your body, and your life.

I wish I could see you a month from now, after you have completed Amy's program. I know you will feel better, with renewed joy and optimism. All best wishes on your journey!

—Felice L. Gersh, MD
   Board Certified in OB/GYN and
   Integrative Medicine;
   Medical Director, Integrative Medical
   Group of Irvine

PART ONE

The PCOS Diva in You

1

Discover Your PCOS Diva

One evening about ten years ago, my husband and I were at a steak house for dinner. As I placed my order, I asked our server some questions about the loaded baked potato that came with my meal.

"Does it come with butter?" I inquired.

"No, it comes with margarine," the waitress replied.

"I can't have margarine," I told her. She made a note to substitute butter for the margarine.

"Can I have a sweet potato instead of a white potato?" I continued. She said that would be fine and asked if I wanted cinnamon sugar.

"No, thank you," I said. "I'll have straight cinnamon."

"No, we only have cinnamon sugar," she replied.

This back-and-forth went on for some time, as I tried to order an unadulterated sweet potato and broccoli with olive oil.

As the waitress made her way to the kitchen, my then clearly irritated husband, Cliff, posed the question that launched PCOS Diva: "When did you become such a diva?"

His question was certainly blunt, and it stung a little, but he was right: I was being a diva.

In that moment, a light went on. What I wish I'd known throughout my journey with polycystic ovary syndrome (PCOS) finally clicked—I deserve to be a PCOS Diva. I need to be a PCOS Diva.

What Is a PCOS Diva?

A PCOS Diva is a woman with hope. She has taken charge of her health and happiness and takes steps every day to enhance both. She chooses to *thrive* with PCOS and is empowered by the knowledge she gathers as she educates herself about PCOS. As a result of her regimen, she is able to give her best to herself and others and be an example of the power of self-care. She is capable of advocating for herself and surrounds herself with the supportive health-care team and community of friends and family she deserves. A PCOS Diva looks beyond the physical support required to manage symptoms and works to heal and enhance her whole person—mind, body, and spirit. A PCOS Diva is an inspiration.

Becoming a PCOS Diva doesn't happen overnight. The journey of healing is lifelong. Every day, a PCOS Diva listens to her body's signals and adjusts her diet and lifestyle, so that she can work in partnership with her body instead of fighting against it.

My path to becoming a PCOS Diva was long and winding. In high school and college, I struggled with hair loss, abnormal hair growth, stress, acne, insulin resistance, weight-loss resistance, and irregular menstrual cycles. I binge-ate and then punished myself with exercise. I could never get a straight answer from health-care professionals about the root cause of my symptoms or how to resolve them. I grew frustrated and hopeless.

It took me fifteen years to get a diagnosis of PCOS and years more to develop a holistic lifestyle plan that's easy, effective, and enjoyable. Today, at age forty-six, I feel stronger, healthier, and more hopeful than ever before. What's more, despite the common misconception that PCOS causes irreversible infertility, I have given birth to three beautiful children, the last conceived naturally after adopting the PCOS Diva lifestyle.

And I'm not alone. Thousands of other women who have followed my programs can attest to my approach's effectiveness. By following an anti-inflammatory diet that's rich in whole foods and mindful indulgences, prioritizing moderate exercise and self-care, and building a support system inside and outside the home, we've learned how to *thrive*, not just survive, with PCOS.

Congratulations! You have taken the first step toward becoming a PCOS Diva. Knowledge is power, and this book will help you develop a diet and lifestyle that work specifically for you. Soon you will be a PCOS Diva too.

The PCOS Diva Difference

The Healing PCOS 21-Day Plan is not a diet plan. If you have been diagnosed with PCOS, then your doctor has likely told you to exercise and lose weight. He or she may have prescribed a pharmaceutical or two as well and sent you on your way. For most women, this approach to treating PCOS doesn't create true, sustainable healing, and there is a good reason for that. It isn't that simple.

Sustainable healing with PCOS cannot be achieved by taking a pill, adopting a low-carb diet, and going to the gym. Healing takes so much more. We need to connect with our bodies and ourselves in a more loving way and learn to think like a PCOS Diva. Only then will we be able to willingly and joyfully make the small, day-to-day diet and lifestyle choices that heal our bodies *and* our minds and souls for a lifetime.

Healing from the inside out is the heart of the PCOS Diva difference. We thrive as a result of self-love and gratitude, not as a result of a trendy, temporary, and unsustainable diet.

Week One: Discover Your PCOS Diva

In Week One, you will discover your PCOS Diva by exploring the foundation of the 21-Day Plan—the way you think about your body, PCOS, and the way you eat. You will discover exactly what works for *you*. No two PCOS Divas are exactly alike, so you will learn to translate your body's unique signals and work in partnership with it.

THINK LIKE A PCOS DIVA

We will begin by changing the way you think about PCOS and your body. Surprised? Many of my clients are shocked that the first thing we do isn't talking about their diet. They expect lists of foods to eat and not to eat right out of the gate. Here's the thing: until you *think* like a PCOS Diva, you cannot *live* like a PCOS Diva. You may make changes that last a few weeks. You may even start to feel a little better. But until you upgrade your thinking, nothing will stick.

In the long run, no drug, diet, or exercise will help you until you take this step. For many women, this is the biggest challenge. It may be easier to pass up a bagel than to look in the mirror and say something nice or prioritize your well-being over someone else's wants.

So we begin by establishing your PCOS Diva mindset and practicing mindfulness. We will work together to develop a perspective that will drive every decision you make, from what to eat to how to deal with stress. Finally, you will learn how to use gratitude to fuel your journey. Over the next 21 days, we will cultivate these elements of your upgraded mindset:

Control: By the end of this transformative 21-day plan, you will have the tools you need to take control of your symptoms and environment instead of playing the role of helpless victim.

Partnering: Your body is not betraying you; it is calling for help. You will learn how to stop fighting your body and instead work

"With PCOS Diva, I learned how important it is to care for me. I realized that if one of my children or my husband had PCOS, I would have been doing this program long ago. I would tirelessly research what was good for them, and I would do everything I could to help them live their best lives. Why wasn't I willing to do that for me? I thought I was being selfish by taking care of myself. I now know the opposite is true. I was being selfish by not taking care of myself. My family needs me. Now they have a healthy mama, and wife who is energetic and engaged. They love the food I make from the meal plans and are moving with me."

—EMMY DARDICK

in partnership with it to recognize its signals and respond in a loving and nurturing way.

Abundance: You will celebrate the abundance in your life. Instead of blaming situations on items you lack or imperfections in yourself and others, you will approach each day with gratitude. The positivity this brings will give you the strength to make the right choices for you.

Progress: You will work toward progress, not perfection. No one is perfect. You will set reasonable goals and celebrate the small wins.

Mindfulness: Truly savoring and being present in a moment will become a habit that will change your perspective on the world and how you move, eat, and love.

Nurturing: Caring for yourself is not selfish, and it is about to change your life. When you approach your body from a place of self-love and compassion, you are better able to hear the messages it is sending to you. You will respond to those messages in a kind and nurturing way, because you understand that you are worth the investment. You are a priority and deserve to feel good.

Please do not skip straight to the 21-Day Plan. There is important information in Part One! For example, you *must* read and internalize Chapter 3, "Think like a PCOS Diva." It is the key to changing your life, controlling your PCOS, and thriving!

EAT LIKE A PCOS DIVA

During Week One, you'll also think about what you use to fuel your body. I love the expression, "Nothing tastes as good as feeling good feels." Although I believe that to be true, eating like a PCOS Diva is no sacrifice. We heal and nurture our bodies with nourishing foods without denying ourselves pleasure. You will discover that:

Food is medicine. Much of what you need to balance your hormones and soothe your PCOS symptoms can be found in the produce section of your grocery store or farmers' market. You will learn which foods heal you and which foods exacerbate your symptoms.

Your body is sending you messages. Your body is telling you what it needs. Those cravings signal something. You will learn how to partner with your body to translate those signals and give it the nutrients it is asking for. There is no one-size-fits-all diet for PCOS. We will find yours.

Food intolerances, sensitivities, and allergies are at the center of many of your symptoms. You will learn how to detect what is inflaming your body and what is healing it. Do tomatoes give you canker sores? Does bread make you feel foggy? Does dairy cause mucus? Learning which foods to avoid will help you develop your individual protocol for eating like a PCOS Diva.

Preparation is essential. You will learn to set yourself up for success with a few minutes of planning and preparation each day. Preparation will save you from raiding the vending machine at work or skipping your daily walk when you get overwhelmed.

No diet is perfect. Day to day, week to week, an essential nutrient or vitamin may be missing from your diet. Which one is it? Which supplements are right for you? You will learn the supplements that commonly help women with PCOS and how to choose the ones that are right for you.

Indulgence is not an indulgence. Feeling deprived is no way to live, and it certainly is no way to live like a PCOS Diva. You will discover satisfying ways to indulge that will not make you feel lousy later.

Week Two: Live like a PCOS Diva

During Week Two, we add the next building block of the PCOS Diva lifestyle—movement. Truly living like a PCOS Diva is more than just how you think and what you eat. It requires regular, joyful movement. Your body is made to move, and once you are in the right mindset and your diet is helping to boost your energy, you will be inspired to move it!

MOVE LIKE A PCOS DIVA

No, this is not where you order a chaise longue to be carried about like Mariah Carey. We are not that kind of diva.

PCOS Divas know how to move joyfully. We understand that regular movement is an important part of the PCOS Diva lifestyle, but we do not punish ourselves with exercise. I cannot count the number of hours I spent on the treadmill, miserably trying to work off calories. Years later, I understand that by approaching exercise as an exhausting chore, I was hurting myself more than I was helping. Not only had overexercising exhausted my adrenal glands and made my symptoms worse; constantly punishing myself was emotionally taxing.

Most women I work with are in the same boat. Exercise is not joyful for them. Does this sound like you too? If it does, I'll help you to find movement you enjoy and *want* to do regularly—and not because you are afraid of the consequences of skipping it. You deserve to feel great and take pleasure in your body and all it can do. You will discover:

The best movement for women with PCOS is . . . whatever you enjoy! Some of the best choices for our metabolism and hormones include high-intensity interval training (HIIT), yoga, and strength training, but the possibilities are endless.

Adrenal fatigue may be keeping you from reaching your goals. Women with PCOS are hormonally vulnerable. Overtaxing our adrenal glands, producers of hormones that control fertility and the stress response, with the wrong types of movement can throw everything out of balance.

The best way to overcome gym anxiety is to think like a PCOS Diva. There is no need to wait until you have a perfect body or lose 10 pounds to go to the gym. You will enjoy going to the gym because it is an act of self-love. Trust me.

Movement and exercise are not weapons to wield against your body. The gym is not a battleground. I know that finding movement you enjoy can be frustrating and even embarrassing. But you can do it, and before you know it, you will be moving like a PCOS Diva (and loving it)!

Week Three: Thrive like a PCOS Diva

During Weeks One and Two, we explore the basics of the PCOS Diva lifestyle and experiment with what works best for you. In Week Three, we add meditation to your daily regimen. At this point, you are ready to step out on your own and practice making your own schedules and menus. You will combine everything you've learned into a sustainable, mindful, and joyful lifestyle tailored just for you. You will discover that:

Meditation benefits the mind and body. Not only does meditation help to calm your mind and ease stress; it has physical benefits all over the body.

There are many ways to meditate. You don't have to do tai chi or chant "Om." You can meditate anytime, anywhere. There's even an app for that.

There is a balance that is optimal for your life. Diet, career, movement, relationships—you juggle all of these things and more. The trick is to find a balance of all these elements. We will use the Thrive like a PCOS Diva Wheel to help find your balance.

Clutter creates chaos. Whether it is piles of stuff on your counters, thoughts racing through your mind, or relationships that don't benefit you, clutter bogs you down. You will learn to clear this clutter and thrive.

This may seem overwhelming, but remember: "Small hinges swing big doors." Becoming healthy isn't going to happen overnight. However, by taking small steps, you can begin to heal your mind and body.

Your Transformation Begins Now

You are ready. The time to partner with your body and take control of your PCOS is now.

I can't wait to start this journey with you. You will not believe the positive impact the changes you will be making over the next three weeks will have on you and even those around you. In fact, you will notice the benefits in as little as a week, but they can last a lifetime. Let's get started!

2

Why You Feel Lousy

As early as age fourteen, I wrestled with many common PCOS symptoms such as acne, hypoglycemia, irregular periods, fatigue, scalp hair loss, and unwanted hair, especially on my face. I wasn't alone. My mother and both grandmothers had similar struggles. It seemed to be the genetic fate of women in my family. Unfortunately, no one was diagnosed with PCOS, so we didn't know there was a root cause for all of these symptoms.

My mother took me to a general practitioner, a dermatologist, a gynecologist, and even a psychologist, and I was subjected to countless tests including a scalp biopsy, yet I had no diagnosis. Not one doctor thought to check my androgens, insulin, or blood sugar. Still, I took the doctors' advice, filled prescriptions, and followed orders. I felt like a victim of my genetics, destined to struggle to get pregnant and some days just to get off the couch. That is, until I chose to take control of my health.

Looking back, I am grateful for my journey. It has shaped the woman that I am and enabled me to help tens of thousands of other women to thrive with PCOS as well. But it was a long journey.

I remember clearly one day in college, when I found myself sitting in a cold medical exam room scared and confused, feeling lousy, not having had a period in months and months, and not understanding why. The doctor looked me in the eye and told me they would have to "jump through hoops" to get me pregnant one day. She renewed my prescription for the pill and sent me on my way. It was a dark moment. I felt helpless and hopeless. I still had no diagnosis. There was no end in sight for my out-of-control symptoms, and now I was facing infertility. Through my twenties, my symptoms worsened. I struck out on my own after college, and that meant eating a lot of inexpensive prepared foods like pasta and macaroni and cheese. I began to struggle with depression. I wondered what was wrong with me. I was a strong, successful, and intelligent woman. Why could I not stop myself from eating Tootsie Rolls? Why was my hair falling out? I was running every day without fail and still gaining weight. I visited an endocrinologist, who gave me spironolactone for my hirsutism (male-pattern hair growth), which did not help because it was only an attempt to treat a symptom. I still didn't receive a diagnosis.

Eventually, I married the love of my life. We wanted to start a family, so I stopped taking the pill. My health struggles and symptoms continued, but four years later, with the help of clomiphene (Clomid), I became pregnant with my first son. He felt like a miracle. After his birth, we decided to try the Creighton Model for family planning, because I didn't want to go back on the pill. I met monthly with a Creighton Model teacher who reviewed my charting, and she soon realized that I was not ovulating. She was the first to notice my patterns and mention PCOS. When we were ready to try for a second child, she referred me to a specialist who put me on Actos, guaifenesin, and Clomid. As with all prescriptions up to this point, I took them without question. No dice. I didn't become pregnant, and I felt awful.

Then I searched out a reproductive endocrinologist. She knew the right labs to request and immediately ordered an ultrasound. Finally! At age thirty, I had my official diagnosis—PCOS. I was put on metformin (which made me horribly sick) and monitored cycles of Clomid. With this help, I conceived my second miracle.

After the birth of my second son, I felt worse than ever. I swore I would never go back on metformin or the pill because both made me feel so awful. I had two beautiful children and a wonderful husband, but I was exhausted all the time and could barely function. My fatigue, hirsutism, brain fog, and hypoglycemia were out of control. I certainly wasn't the wife or mother I knew I could be. After years of following mainstream advice from countless doctors, I realized that nothing was helping. The drugs they offered made me sicker and more miserable. The drugs that helped get me pregnant couldn't heal my PCOS. I was way too young to feel so old, and sick and tired of feeling sick and tired—I couldn't go on living this way.

I knew that if I wanted to feel better, I had to adopt a different approach. I found a naturopath to help me get to the root of my symptoms instead of trying to put a Band-Aid on each one. At thirty-two years old, I found the right person. She guided me in selecting supplements that could naturally balance my hormones. Maybe most important, she taught me to how to use a glucometer. Thanks to this tool, I made the connection between what I was eating and how I was feeling. I had empirical evidence to help make sense of my symptoms. Glucometer in hand, I began to experiment with my diet. As I mastered this piece of my life, my energy returned, my hair slowly began to grow back, I lost weight, and my menstrual cycles began to regulate.

In working with my naturopath and doing my own research and experimentation, I realized that I had the power to take control of my health. No one else could do it for me. I couldn't take advice at face value and continue to think and act like a victim.

I scoured the internet for information and read books about PCOS and holistic medicine by pioneers like Samuel Thatcher, Walter Futterweit, and Nancy Dunne. I went back to school to learn from experts about nutrition and healing. After hundreds of hours and tons of trial and error, I developed a protocol that allowed me to thrive. I changed my diet and lifestyle and, most important, my mindset. I started taking care of myself. My husband noticed the shift and declared me a "diva." At first, I was offended, until I realized that in order to be my best and give my best to my family, I did have to be a PCOS Diva.

When my reproductive endocrinologist started seeing my success and sending women with PCOS who also couldn't tolerate metformin or the pill to me for help, I knew I was onto something. I received my health-coaching certificate and began to formally coach women one-on-one with great success. Soon I realized that the small, manageable *steps of what is now my Healing PCOS 21-Day Plan could help the millions of other women struggling to alleviate their symptoms with medicine and advice that didn't help. Now sharing what I know about PCOS is my passion and career. And, despite what doctors warned all those years ago, I conceived my third child, an amazing girl, naturally. She's the direct product of the PCOS Diva lifestyle I forged.*

I want you to know that you are not a victim. Struggling with PCOS is not your fate. There is no magic pill, but you can thrive with PCOS when you embrace the power of knowledge, diet, and lifestyle.

What Is Polycystic Ovary Syndrome (PCOS)?

You are not alone. Polycystic ovary syndrome (PCOS) is one of the most common endocrine system disorders found in women and the most common cause of infertility in women. As calculated employing the widely used Rotterdam Criteria, PCOS affects approximately 15 to 20 percent of women worldwide, of whom less than 50 percent are diagnosed. It is present throughout a woman's life from puberty through postmenopause and affects women of all races and ethnic groups.

As an endocrine disorder, PCOS disrupts hormone balance, negatively impacting many bodily functions including insulin levels, cell and tissue growth and development, metabolism, fertility, and cognition. A diagnosis is often difficult to obtain because PCOS is a syndrome, a collection of symptoms. It affects many different hormones, resulting in an array of symptoms that may seem unrelated and vary from woman to woman. Some symptoms include obesity, irregular menstrual cycles, insulin resistance, infertility, depression, male-pattern hair growth, acne, and hair loss.

In addition, women with PCOS have a four to seven times higher risk of heart attack, and 50 percent will develop prediabetes or diabetes before age forty. They are also more likely to develop endometrial cancer. The increased risk of these serious health issues makes managing symptoms even more imperative—and stressful.

——————— What Are the Symptoms of PCOS? ———————

You may have one or two of these symptoms or a dozen. Although some symptoms are more common than others, there is no single model for PCOS.

- Oligoovulation (irregular ovulation) or anovulation (absent ovulation)

- Polycystic ovaries

- High levels of insulin, insulin resistance (30–50 percent)

- Easy weight gain and/or obesity (55–80 percent)

- Fertility issues

- Acne (40–60 percent)

- Cardiovascular issues

- Type 2 diabetes

- Depression (28–64 percent)

- Anxiety (34–57 percent)

- Poor body image, eating disorders (21 percent)

- Sexual dysfunction

- Thyroid disorders

- High levels of androgens (60–80 percent)

- Irregular menstruation (75–80 percent)

- Male-pattern hair growth (70 percent)

- Skin tags

- Sleep apnea (8 percent)

- Gray-white breast discharge (8–10 percent)

- Scalp hair loss (40–70 percent)

- Darkening skin areas (acanthosis nigricans), particularly on the nape of the neck (10 percent)

- Pelvic pain

- Hidradenitis suppurativa (painful boil-like abscesses in the groin)

Some of the Most Common Symptoms

The most common symptoms of PCOS are insulin resistance and hyperinsulinemia, hormone imbalances, and chronic inflammation.

INSULIN RESISTANCE AND HYPERINSULINEMIA

Insulin resistance, when cells fail to respond normally to the hormone insulin, and *hyperinsulinemia*, chronically high levels of insulin in the blood, are both symptoms with which I struggled all my life. Unfortunately, as is probably the case with many of you, they went undiagnosed for many years.

I remember fainting multiple times in sixth grade. The nurse didn't know what was wrong. My mom took me to doctors, who also found nothing and finally referred me for psychiatric evaluation. Imagine being twelve years old, feeling horrible, and being told it is all in your head. Many years later, still undiagnosed, I remember feeling baffled when every Sunday morning, after my fiancé and I had our traditional waffle breakfast complete with syrup and orange juice, I would get woozy in church. Little did I know, it was the waffle breakfast throwing my blood sugar out of whack and giving me hypoglycemia! Since then, I have learned to interpret my body's signals. Now when I feel that way, I know exactly what to do.

Insulin resistance and hyperinsulinemia are conditions in which the body becomes less and less efficient at processing and managing levels of sugar (glucose) in the bloodstream. This has serious overall health consequences. In the short term, insulin resistance is at the heart of most PCOS symptoms, including infertility, obesity, hirsutism, hyperandrogenism (elevated androgen levels), chronic fatigue syndrome, immune system defects, eating disorders, hypoglycemia, gastrointestinal disorders, depression, and anxiety. In the long term, when insulin levels rise too high, type 2 diabetes may result. Hardening of the

Symptoms of Insulin Resistance

- Weight gain
- Sugar cravings
- Skin tags
- Hypoglycemia
- Rough or red bumps on upper arms
- Dark skin patches on neck, knees, elbows, knuckles, chest, or groin

arteries (atherosclerosis) is a common result of insulin dysfunction and may lead to an increased risk of high blood pressure and stroke.

In a healthy system, insulin plays an important role in metabolism. This powerful hormone is produced by the pancreas and enters the bloodstream after a meal. Its main function is to transport glucose to cells throughout the body to be used for energy. When there is excess glucose, insulin delivers the glucose to muscles, fat, and the liver, which helps to lower the blood glucose levels by storing it and signaling the body to slow production of insulin. But in an unhealthy system, insulin resistance and hyperinsulinemia may result.

Between 50 and 70 percent of women with PCOS have some degree of insulin resistance. Insulin resistance may be caused by poor diet, ethnicity, certain diseases, hormones, steroid use, some medications, older age, sleep problems, and cigarette smoking. Although insulin resistance is often associated with obesity, research indicates that lean PCOS patients are also prone to insulin resistance. Research also indicates that the birth control pill may cause insulin resistance in all women, particularly those with PCOS.

Insulin resistance occurs when a person's body does not react properly to the amount of insulin in the bloodstream. In a healthy system, after a meal, the pancreas creates insulin to balance the glucose in the blood. Ideally, the body detects if the level of glucose in the blood is still too high and signals the pancreas to create more insulin. The hope is that since there is more insulin, more glucose will be picked up.

Insulin in large quantities can be toxic to cells, so when there is too much insulin in the body over time, cells become insulin resistant in order to protect themselves. Alternatively, the hypothalamus may become insulin resistant and continue to send signals to the pancreas to create more insulin unnecessarily. When insulin resistance occurs, the insulin does not pick up or cannot deliver the glucose to the cells that need it. Glucose levels in the blood remain high, and diabetes and other serious health disorders may result.

Hyperinsulinemia results when more insulin is present in the bloodstream than is considered normal, usually as a result of insulin resistance. Although it is associated with diabetes, someone with hyperinsulinemia does not necessarily have diabetes.

Insulin resistance and hyperinsulinemia create a self-perpetuating and destructive cycle called the *insulin resistance cycle*. Insulin resistance creates chronically high levels of insulin, and those chronically high levels bombard cells, forcing them to protect themselves, thus perpetuating insulin resistance. Eventually, your pancreas can no longer keep up with the insulin demand. This means there is less insulin in the body to store and regulate glucose levels, and the result is diabetes.

In addition, high levels of insulin and insulin resistance sometimes pave the way for hyperandrogenism, excessive levels of male hormones. This may be the cause of missed periods and infertility in some women with PCOS. The relationship between hyperandrogenism and hyperinsulinemia in women with PCOS is unclear. Researchers disagree about whether hyperinsulinemia causes hyperandrogenism, hyperandrogenism causes hyperinsulinemia, or a third cause is responsible for both. One way or the other, we have a destructive cycle: insulin resistance leads to hyperandrogenism, which increases insulin levels.

A top priority of the Healing PCOS 21-Day Plan is to get your insulin under control.

HORMONE IMBALANCES

When my hair started falling out during high school, my mom took me to a dermatologist who did a scalp biopsy. When it came back negative, the hair loss as well as other symptoms such as fatigue, acne, and sporadic periods were written off as a result of stress. Things got worse as I grew older. I began gaining weight, growing facial hair, experiencing anxiety and depression, and still fighting the symptoms I had since puberty. The birth control pill that was supposed to be my "quick fix" manipulated my hormones, leaving me feeling moody and dull. I wish that I had had a better understanding then of how my hormones work and how hormone imbalances caused by diet and lifestyle choices could be the source of my symptoms.

Hormones are responsible for keeping your major bodily functions running smoothly, so when hormone levels become imbalanced, you'll feel the effects in many ways. Hirsutism, acne, hair loss, higher stress levels, mood disorders, depression, anxiety, and infertility can all result.

The most common hormones that become imbalanced and the ones that you will learn to manage with the Healing PCOS 21-Day Plan are androgens, cortisol, progesterone, estrogen, and thyroid hormones.

Androgens: Androgens are male hormones, such as testosterone, dihydrotestosterone (DHT), dehydroepiandrosterone (DHEA), and DHEA sulfate (DHEA-S). In males, these steroid hormones are responsible for sexual development and muscle mass. In women, they play a much subtler, though no less important role. Among other things, they help us maintain muscle mass, regulate our weight, and keep our libidos humming. They are produced in the ovaries, adrenal glands, and fat cells. The problem isn't that women with PCOS have androgens; it is that we typically have an excess. This androgen excess, or hyperandrogenism, affects about 25 percent of women with PCOS and is often the root cause of common symptoms such as hirsutism, acne, hair loss, and infertility.

Androgen excess may be caused by:

- Ovarian dysfunction, which causes the ovaries to produce excess testosterone.
- Insulin resistance, which signals the ovaries to produce excess testosterone.

- Stress, which taxes the adrenal glands and stimulates the production of androgen hormones. For this reason, women with PCOS should practice stress relief from an early age.
- Early adrenal activation, which initiates early puberty and correlates with increased lifelong androgen formation. Girls who experience early puberty may have an increased risk of developing PCOS.
- Obesity.
- Genetics.
- Taking artificial hormones in birth control.
- Individual hypersensitivity to a normal amount of androgen.
- A defect in the hypothalamus, a part of the brain responsible for regulating the production of many hormones, including androgens.

Cortisol: Women with PCOS often make too much cortisol, the "stress hormone" produced in the adrenal glands. In fact, research indicates that many women with PCOS may naturally have higher cortisol levels. Being overweight also increases cortisol production.

Raised levels of cortisol change the way your body manages other critical hormones, putting you at risk for insulin resistance, anxiety, depression, and thyroid dysfunction. In addition, the overproduction of cortisol can overwork the adrenals to the point of adrenal fatigue. For this reason, stress—emotional or physical—takes more of a toll on women with PCOS than on those without it.

Progesterone: Progesterone is a hormone, produced mainly in the ovaries, that plays an important role in the menstrual cycle and maintaining and nourishing the body during pregnancy. After ovulation each month, progesterone helps thicken the uterine lining in preparation for a fertilized egg. This is called the luteal phase of the menstrual cycle. Women with PCOS almost always have low progesterone and thus a luteal-phase defect. This makes it nearly impossible to maintain a pregnancy even if ovulation and implantation do occur and is often the cause of miscarriage and unsuccessful assisted reproduction. Some doctors recommend supplemental progesterone for women with

————————— Signs of Low Progesterone —————————

- Anxiety
- Waking at night
- Fibrocystic breasts
- PMS
- Bone loss
- Low libido
- Infertility or irregular periods

PCOS in order to support early pregnancy if they have suffered multiple miscarriages.

If you have a progesterone deficiency and your doctor suggests hormone replacement, you may be prescribed a bioidentical progesterone. Bioidentical, or natural, progesterone is a combination of elements derived from natural plant sources that identically matches the progesterone we naturally make in our bodies. Prometrium is a micronized (reduced to tiny particles and mixed with peanut oil) natural progesterone in the form of a pill. It is approved by the Food and Drug Administration (FDA) as a natural hormone-replacement therapy medication. Because natural progesterone is molecularly identical to the hormone produced by the body, it causes few side effects.

Alternatively, your doctor may suggest a synthetic progestin such as Provera, since it was the standard before good natural alternatives were developed. Provera is also a constructed compound, but its chemical structure is not identical to natural progesterone. As a result, it can cause changes in vaginal bleeding, blood sugar issues, blood clots, and depression. Unfortunately, many women are told that synthetic progestin is the same as natural progesterone. Be a PCOS Diva at the doctor's office and discuss the differences between these two hormone-replacement options to find one that is best for you.

Estrogen: Estrogen, the primary female sex hormone, is produced in the ovaries, adrenal glands, and fat tissues. Many women with PCOS

Signs of Estrogen Dominance

- PMS
- Headaches and/or migraines
- Fluid retention
- Heavy or painful periods
- Endometriosis
- Moodiness, anxiety, or depression
- Hypothyroidism
- Infertility or miscarriage
- Breast pain or tenderness

experience estrogen dominance, that is, too much estrogen and not enough progesterone to balance its effects. Symptoms such as heavy or painful periods, infertility/miscarriage, and hypothyroidism (an underactive thyroid gland) may result.

Thyroid hormones: Many women with PCOS have a dysfunctional thyroid. It may be overactive (hyperthyroidism) or, more commonly, underactive (hypothyroidism). Hashimoto's disease, an autoimmune disease and the most common cause of hypothyroidism, is prevalent in women with PCOS.

If the thyroid is not functioning properly, the balance of thyroid hormones and every other hormone in the body will be disrupted,

"Think of PCOS as being in an extended state of puberty, where androgens, luteinizing hormone (LH), and insulin resistance dominate and follicle-stimulating hormone (FSH), estrogen, and progesterone haven't established their rhythm."

—DR. FIONA MCCULLOCH

causing abnormal sexual development, menstrual irregularities, and possibly infertility. I encourage all women with PCOS symptoms to have a complete set of thyroid labs to rule out thyroid dysfunction.

───────────   Signs of Thyroid Dysfunction   ───────────

Signs of Hypothyroidism (Underactive Thyroid)

- Unexplained weight gain or trouble losing weight
- Fatigue
- Depression
- Hair loss and dry hair
- Muscle cramps
- Dry skin
- Swelling of the thyroid gland
- Brittle nails
- Slow heart rate
- Irregular period
- Sensitivity to cold
- Constipation

Signs of Hyperthyroidism (Overactive Thyroid)

- Unexplained weight loss
- Palpitations
- Feeling wired or anxious
- Shakiness
- Sweating spells
- Feeling hot frequently
- Tremors
- Shortness of breath
- Itchy red skin
- More frequent bowel movements than usual
- Fine hair and hair loss

CHRONIC INFLAMMATION

*I should be a dentist's dream patient. My brushing and flossing habits
are impeccable. I have my teeth cleaned every six months. I don't poke
around in my mouth with pointy objects. Then why did my gums
bleed every time I went to the dentist? For years, no matter what I
tried, from my dentist I would get that face and "the talk." You know
the one I mean, about brushing and flossing regularly? As it turns out,
it wasn't my oral hygiene that was the problem. It was my systemic
inflammation.*

Inflammation isn't necessarily bad. Our bodies use inflammation to
fight off microbial, autoimmune, metabolic, or physical attacks. For
example, it's what causes our knees to puff up and bleed when we fall
and scrape them. It's a sign the body is deploying white blood cells,

─────────── Symptoms of Inflammation ───────────

- Weight gain
- Allergies
- Brain fog
- Joint pain
- Irritable bowel syndrome
- GI issues (bloating, gas, diarrhea)
- Acne
- Asthma
- Gum disease
- Chronic sinusitis
- High blood sugar
- Depression
- Belly fat
- Fatigue
- Eczema
- Psoriasis

which help heal injuries, fend off disease, and replace aging cells. The problem is chronic inflammation, inflammation lasting from a few months to several years. That type of inflammation takes a tremendous toll on every system of the body.

According to integrative physician Felice Gersh, chronic inflammation is the root cause of many of the conditions women with PCOS experience, such as obesity and weight-loss resistance, infertility, hirsutism, mood swings, and acne. And recent research suggests that women with PCOS have higher levels of circulating C-reactive protein (CRP), an indicator of general inflammation independent even of obesity.

Inflammation is widely recognized as the root of many of the major diseases that plague the Western world. Cardiovascular disease, metabolic syndrome, hypertension, some cancers, diabetes, and PCOS all share the common root of inflammation.

Chronic inflammation may be caused by obesity, food sensitivities and allergies, and stress. It may also result from environmental and lifestyle factors such as pollution, poor diet, smoking, lack of exercise, and poor dental health. Getting to the root of these problems through a proper inflammation-reducing diet and lifestyle is critical for women with PCOS.

Why Do I Have PCOS?

Although the exact cause of PCOS is unknown, it is generally agreed that genetics, hyperinsulinemia (high levels of insulin) and insulin resistance, and/or a defect in a hormone-producing organ play a role. I have already discussed the chicken-and-egg debate about insulin and PCOS, whether chronically high levels of insulin cause excess androgens or vice versa. With regard to genetics, studies show that a woman with PCOS has a 40 percent likelihood of having a sister with the syndrome and a 35 percent chance of having a mother with the disorder. It is possible that a mother's obesity, insulin resistance, or exposure to food high in advanced glycation end products (AGEs) or industrial toxins such as bisphenol A (BPA) may be the root cause. If PCOS is genetic, the genes involved in its expression may be triggered by environmental stimuli such as poor diet or rapid weight gain.

Some women with PCOS first experience symptoms when they stop taking the birth control pill. Typically, there was a predisposition before taking the pill, but only when they stopped taking it did symptoms emerge as a result of the disruption in communication between the pituitary gland and ovaries. In this case, symptoms should clear as soon as communication is reestablished.

How Can I Get Diagnosed?

Getting a firm diagnosis can be a long journey. There are several things to remember when seeking a diagnosis:

Be honest with your doctors. Tell them all of your symptoms. Try not to be embarrassed, and don't write symptoms off to genetics, saying something like, "My aunts all have thinning hair; it must be genetic." Your aunts may all have PCOS!

PCOS has a name problem. Approximately 20 percent of women who do *not* have PCOS have cysts on their ovaries. Similarly, about 30 percent of women who do have PCOS have *no* cysts.

Doctors are not always well-educated about PCOS and may try to treat each symptom separately instead of looking for the root cause. Press to get to the heart of your symptoms.

Be assertive when asking for lab tests. The more information you and your doctor can collect, the quicker you will get to the root of your symptoms and develop an effective plan. For a complete list of suggested labs, visit PCOSDiva.com/labs.

There is no definitive test to determine whether you have PCOS, but the most widely accepted diagnostic criteria are the Rotterdam Criteria. These were developed by the European Society for Human Reproduction and the American Society for Reproductive Medicine and include the original National Institutes of Health and EAE-PCOS Society diagnostic criteria. To be diagnosed with PCOS, a woman must present two of these three criteria:

1. Oligoovulation (irregular ovulation) or anovulation (absent ovulation)
2. Hyperandrogenism (elevated levels of androgenic hormones such as testosterone, clinical and/or biochemical)
3. Polycystic ovaries (enlarged ovaries containing at least twelve follicles each, shown on an ultrasound)

Even with these criteria in place, diagnosis can be tricky. Medications like birth control pills alter androgen levels and make testing inaccurate. Keep in mind that women may have irregular or even regular cycles and not ovulate or only ovulate occasionally. Having a period does not mean that you are ovulating. In addition, the presentation of symptoms may vary. There is no one-size-fits-all characterization of PCOS. You may be overweight and have irregular periods and acne, and the next woman may be lean with polycystic ovaries, absent periods, and hirsutism.

It is possible that you do not meet the Rotterdam Criteria at all, but still suffer from the symptoms. PCOS is often used as an umbrella term to include women with similar symptoms stemming from hyperandrogenism. You may also have a thyroid condition, and, again, I encourage all women with PCOS symptoms to have a complete set of thyroid labs to rule out thyroid dysfunction. You may have post-pill PCOS, a temporary condition with many of the same symptoms as PCOS caused by coming off of the birth control pill. If this is the case, once you rebalance your hormones, your symptoms should clear up for good.

As you can see, no single treatment will work for all women. The Healing PCOS 21-Day Plan is designed so that you can examine your symptoms, find the root cause, and discover what works for *you*.

Why Medications May Not Help:
The "Band-Aid Effect"

I hear from women every day whose PCOS journeys had a very similar beginning. In their teens, they had irregular periods, acne, and/or painful PMS. Their doctor "fixed" these symptoms by prescribing the pill. Now the journeys divide. Some women tolerated the pill, but when they got off it, their symptoms returned with a vengeance and they struggled to conceive. Others could not tolerate the pill (nausea, headaches, weight gain, loss of libido) and have struggled with their symptoms and a series of drugs meant to help ever since.

There is a reason that these drugs cannot provide real, sustainable healing. At best, they are nothing more than Band-Aids, covering symptoms but not treating the root cause. At worst, they complicate your health picture with destructive side effects.

The Birth Control Pill

The pill is hands-down the go-to prescription from doctors. It has been touted as a miracle drug for everything from regulating periods to clearing up acne. In many cases, it seems to work for a while, but eventually you stop taking it and your symptoms return. Unfortunately, the pill has some serious downsides that most women are never told about.

- **Blood clots.** Research indicates that women on the birth control pill increase their risk of blood clots by a factor of 1.6. For those taking pills with higher levels of estrogen, that risk is twice as high. This risk throws fuel on the fire for women with PCOS who are already at higher risk for heart attacks and stroke.
- **Increased insulin resistance.** Studies show that with certain types of birth control pills, women suffered "unfavorable changes of insulin sensitivity." This was certainly my experience. Researchers believe that this may have to do with the ratio of estrogen and progestin used in the various pills. Due to this concern about estrogen and insulin resistance, many doctors do

not prescribe the pill for women at risk for or who already have diabetes. Whatever the reason, women with PCOS should not be taking any medications that worsen insulin resistance.

- **Lower libido.** The pill, by definition, alters your hormones. Unfortunately, for some women, it dampens libido (you see the irony). This happens for a couple of reasons. First, the steady stream of synthetic hormones from the pill evens out the body's natural cycle of high (around ovulation) and low libido. Second, it suppresses testosterone levels. That's great for taking care of androgen-induced symptoms (acne, facial hair), but is lousy for your sex drive.

- **Nutrient deficiency.** The pill depletes levels of valuable nutrients such as B vitamins, folic acid, vitamins C and E, magnesium, and zinc. You need sufficient levels of zinc to maintain a healthy hormone balance. Weight gain, fluid retention, mood changes, depression, and even heart disease can all arise from nutrient imbalance.

- **Candida.** Estrogen promotes the growth of yeast in the gut, sometimes causing a condition called *Candida* overgrowth. *Candida* is a fungus (a form of yeast) that occurs naturally in small amounts and aids in digestion. If an overgrowth occurs, symptoms like brain fog, fatigue, digestive and skin issues, mood swings, and fungal infections occur. In addition, it breaks through the intestinal wall and allows byproducts into the surrounding area, triggering systemic inflammation. Since the major ingredient in the pill is estrogen, the risk of *Candida* overgrowth increases; it also causes sugar and carb cravings.

Metformin

After the birth control pill, metformin is the most commonly pre-scribed drug to "treat" PCOS. The purpose of metformin is to de-crease the amount of glucose (sugar) and insulin produced by the liver and pancreas, and increase sensitivity to insulin in muscle cells. Getting insulin resistance under control is critical to thriving with PCOS, so it makes sense to take a pill and get quick results, right? Unfortunately, according to a National Institutes of Health 2012 study: "Metformin decreases androgen levels but has demonstrated only modest effect on fertility and has little effect on insulin action." Here are a few of the problems with metformin:

- **GI issues.** Metformin doesn't only work in the liver; it takes action in the gut. It effectively adds to the protective mucus layer and stimulates pathways for fat burning and cellular rejuvenation, which should lead to more effective glucose regulation. In the process, many women (like me) find that it causes more GI distress (nausea, cramping, diarrhea) than it is worth.
- **Nutrient depletion.** Metformin is widely acknowledged to deplete vitamin B_{12}. A shortage of B_{12} is associated with nerve pain (neuropathy), cognitive dysfunction, and anemias.
- **Band-Aid effect.** Like so many medications, metformin does not fix the underlying problem. Poor diet and lifestyle choices are usually the root of insulin resistance. Failure to change those will limit the effectiveness of this drug, and if it is ever stopped, the symptoms will return.

Spironolactone

Spironolactone (Aldactone) is a diuretic often prescribed to treat symptoms associated with high levels of androgens such as acne, hirsutism, and thinning scalp hair. It is not meant to treat insulin resistance, the cause of high levels of androgens in women with PCOS. Reducing the level of androgens in the body with a pill instead of addressing the root cause is a Band-Aid at best. The moment a woman stops taking the drug, symptoms will return.

Flutamide

Like spironolactone, flutamide works as an anti-androgen. In fact, its intended purpose is to reduce testosterone in the treatment of prostate cancer. In women, it has been found to be an effective drug for treating hirsutism and mild to moderate acne. Some studies indicate it works

Although you cannot cure PCOS, you can manage your symptoms
through diet, exercise, and other lifestyle approaches.

better than spironolactone. Like all of these drugs, flutamide is a Band-
Aid treatment and does not attempt to resolve the root cause of the
condition. In addition, there is risk of serious liver problems and birth
defects if taken when pregnant. In fact, many doctors will not prescribe
flutamide to women at all.

What Can I Do?

So now that you know why you feel lousy, what can you do?

You can heal and thrive! Although you cannot cure PCOS, you can
manage your symptoms through diet, exercise, and other lifestyle approaches. Doctors and researchers agree that lifestyle therapy should be
the first line of treatment for women with PCOS. Managing diet, lifestyle, and emotional health will lead to better health, restore hormonal
balance, and help get your insulin levels back on track. Before you
know it, your symptoms will begin to ease and your risk of diabetes,
heart disease, hypertension, sleep apnea, anxiety, depression, and infertility will decrease. Therefore, a holistic approach is required to tame
the symptoms of PCOS and improve your quality of life. *Above all, we
need to be thoughtful about the foods we use to fuel our bodies, the exercise we
choose, the toxins we are exposed to, and, just as important, the emotional and
mental care we take of ourselves.*

But I Really Just Want to Take a Magic Pill

Good news. There is a magic pill. It's you. The moment you decide
that you deserve to be healthy and happy, you will begin to make
the changes necessary to heal. You will wake up every day and make
choices that nurture yourself, and you will feel better. As you feel better, you will make even more upgrades, and the cycle will continue.
You are the magic pill that makes it all possible.

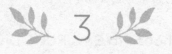

Think like a PCOS Diva

Everyone has a rock bottom. I remember mine clearly. My husband came home from work one day to find me lying on the couch listless and hopeless, my boys, ages four and one, running wild. I could not muster the energy to play with them, these babies I loved so dearly, had wanted so badly, and worked so hard for. My fatigue and other PCOS symptoms had drained the life out of me. I wasn't the mom and wife I wanted to be and knew I could be.

I saw myself through my husband's eyes that afternoon. I saw myself and knew it was time to take control of my health and my life. This woman on the couch was not me. Moreover, I didn't want to be her.

Until that moment, I had followed my doctors' advice. I took the tests they suggested and the drugs they prescribed. But nothing was working. At this "aha" moment, I realized that I had to stop being passive about my care. I needed to take control of it and educate myself about PCOS, so that I could make informed decisions. I needed to become my own advocate, and to do that I knew that I first needed to change my frame of mind. I had to want to feel better; I had to know in my heart that I could heal and that I deserved to feel better. Realizing that I was worth saving changed the way I thought about my life, my body, and my PCOS. *Once my mindset shifted, I began my journey of thriving with PCOS.*

Choose to Be a PCOS Diva

You may be asking yourself why "Think like a PCOS Diva" comes before "Eat like a PCOS Diva." You are wondering why you can't just exercise, eliminate gluten, and be all set. You cannot. Here's why. *If you do not think like a PCOS Diva, you cannot be a PCOS Diva (not for long at least).*

Being a PCOS Diva involves a conscious manner of thinking that is the key to making the PCOS Diva lifestyle sustainable. In order for diet and lifestyle changes to work, you must *believe* that you can feel better and know that you *deserve* to feel better. With this mindset shift, you will eliminate the chance for failure or self-sabotage. When you *expect* to succeed, you will find a way to overcome any minor setback, because you are on your chosen path. Setbacks (although frustrating) become an opportunity to learn.

Imagine it like this. You and your friend are on your way to dinner at a restaurant you've been wanting to try. On the way, you find that

"I have been a PCOS Diva for a year now, and I feel healthy and alive. I actually *want* to go outside and run around with my eleven-year-old, and my relationships have shifted in a huge way. I finally believe in myself and can say for the first time in my life that I feel love and compassion for myself, which allowed me to believe that my husband loved me no matter what. This was a big one for me, because I realized that I had been living my life with the belief that I didn't *deserve* to be loved; not by others or by myself. I feel strong and capable and know that I have control over the whole big picture of PCOS now."

—NICOLE M.

the bridge to get there is washed out. You can still go, but you have to take a detour that adds an hour to your drive. You will likely choose a different restaurant tonight, right? Now imagine that you own that restaurant and it supports your family. You need to be there to open the door for the employees and customers. You will find a way over this obstacle. You will take the detour. Heck, you might build a raft or swim!

If you believe that you must be at your destination, you will find a way. Healing is the same. It is much harder to give up on something you know you deserve, something you must be, something that is a part of you. You will make choices and take actions based on thinking like a PCOS Diva, you will start to feel better, and the PCOS Diva lifestyle will stick for life.

Mastering Your Mindset

The *victim*, *fighting*, and *lack* mindsets frequently hold us back. By upgrading these mindsets to *in control*, *partnering*, and *abundance* we will upgrade your thinking to the PCOS Diva level.

From a Victim to an In-Control Mindset

A victim is someone who has been hurt or taken advantage of by someone or something and feels helpless in the face of the circumstances. I can understand why many women with PCOS feel like victims of their syndrome. I did. Living each day with frustrating and often embarrassing symptoms can wear you down and make you feel helpless. The feeling of helplessness grows when doctors' advice and drugs don't seem to help.

The problem with considering yourself a victim of PCOS is that the very act of deciding you are a victim takes away your power. Victims are powerless against their circumstances. When you decide that you are a victim, you choose not to act and take control. You choose to let circumstances or symptoms "win." You stop looking for solutions.

The fact that you have PCOS isn't your fault. Choosing to be a victim is. Here's the thing: *PCOS Divas are not victims.* We are not powerless. Our bodies have not betrayed us. We are not helpless in the struggle against our symptoms.

Step one to thriving with PCOS is deciding that you *can* thrive with PCOS. So PCOS Divas take control of two things. First, we take control of our mindset and begin to think like a PCOS Diva.

I deserve to feel good.

I take steps to feel better.

I can thrive and live my best life.

I work *with* my body.

I am in control of my PCOS (or at least I am working on it).

Step two is taking control of our body, what we put in it, and how we use it and care for it.

I eat in a way that shows I love my body.

I move in a way that I enjoy and makes me strong.

I seek out knowledge about PCOS and how to heal.

I ask for support.

I don't take the first answer I am given. I research and get second opinions.

I treat my body and mind with love and respect.

"I have never felt better about myself. I sit here crying because I am getting healthy! I am taking my life into my own hands. I am no longer a victim. I do not have to live like everyone else is going to fix it. I see life through new eyes, and I have the ability to choose good things. To choose health. To choose self-care. To choose self-nurture. To choose me."
—NELDA

When you stop playing the victim and take the power into your hands, you make the decisions that make you better. There is no waiting around for things to get better on their own or for a doctor to prescribe a magic pill. You're in charge!

A PCOS Diva is not a victim (feeling hopeless and looking for pity). She is in control (in charge and hopeful).

Good news. You're already embracing an in-control mindset. Choosing to become a PCOS Diva is empowering. Choosing this book was an empowering decision that set you on the right path. You are taking control. You are already on your way!

From now on, you will make a conscious choice every day to be in control of your health, happiness, and PCOS. Positive habits, like eating foods that heal your body, will spring from that choice.

From a Fighting to a Partnering Mindset

Now that you are taking control of your PCOS, it's time to get your mental and physical selves working together. I often hear women say they are "fighting" their symptoms or "conquering" or "battling" PCOS. Let's stop approaching our lives that way. Here's why. When you have symptoms, it is not that your body is fighting or sabotaging you. Symptoms are your body's way of communicating with you. Think of it as your body waving a red flag that something is wrong and asking for help. For example:

Irregular periods ➞ "Our hormones are out of whack. Can we fix this?"

Acne ➞ "We have some inflammation going on. Can we tame these flames?"

Weight gain (especially around the middle) ➞ "Our insulin is way too high. We are processing as fast as we can, but let's get this under control!"

The moment you team up with your body and listen to its signals, you can hear those signals more clearly and soothe the symptoms in a loving way.

Divas take control of their health one step at a time. We know that our bodies are sending us signals about what is wrong and how to fix it. We work hard to tune in to those messages and work in sync. We don't fight ourselves!

From a Lack to an Abundance Mindset

Approaching life from a lack mindset means focusing on the things that don't go our way or what we don't have. Instead, we can consciously choose to approach life from an abundance mindset, celebrating every day's small triumphs and blessings.

Approaching the day from a place of abundance, gratitude, and positivity, looking for the good, changes everything. You will start to feel lighter and your stress levels will fall, and as a result you will begin to feel better. Solutions will present themselves.

"With the guidance of PCOS Diva, I went from feeling that something was wrong with my body, that my body was faulty and not fully feminine due to PCOS, to thriving, having cycles, and having a body that I loved. I followed your guidance and found that inside my body was perfect; it just needed more love, and I needed to be a 'Diva' and to take control of the way I cared for my body. I noticed changes after the first few weeks and have maintained a healthy body and menstrual cycles for three years (after having never had normal cycles in my entire life) at the age of thirty-five."

—JENNIFER R.

Lack Thinking	Abundance Thinking
I will never be enough.	I am enough.
I am judgmental.	I appreciate.
I look for what is going wrong.	I look for what is going right.
I am rigid and closed off from new ideas.	I am open to new ideas.
I am jealous and envious of others.	I celebrate others' success.
I compare myself to others.	I am authentic.
I am a perfectionist.	I focus on progress.
I am fear-based.	I focus on and notice blessings in life.
I never feel that I have enough time or money.	I am generous.
I am a victim of PCOS.	I am in control of my health.

As you learn to be a PCOS Diva, remember this mantra: "Progress, not perfection." As long as you are progressing toward your goal, you are on the right path. Don't wait for life to be perfect before you approach every day with an abundance mindset. There is no perfect. No one has a perfect life—no matter what it looks like on social media. Please do not put your life on hold while you wait to achieve some ideal. Donate those clothes you are waiting to fit back into. Love who you are in this moment, and appreciate what you have. Today, you are enough, you have enough.

It has taken me a long time to embrace "Progress, not perfection." I am a recovering perfectionist. Striving for perfection left me exhausted, frustrated, and feeling bad about myself. Insisting upon perfection was taking a toll on myself and those around me. It was unsustainable. To get healthy, I had to put my perfectionist tendencies aside. I learned that missteps were lessons not failures.

If you are a recovering perfectionist like me, remember, as you move through the Healing PCOS 21-Day Plan, to not strive to do everything perfectly. Do as much as you can. Congratulate yourself on your successes. Learn from your missteps. The more you do, the faster you will feel better, but this is not a race; it's your journey.

Let's be real. This change in thinking doesn't happen overnight. You didn't just read the last two paragraphs and think, "Oh, okay. I am enough. Everything is fine. Phew." Give yourself time to retrain your brain into thinking from an abundance perspective. We will work on this over the next 21 days. Remember, "Progress, not perfection."

PCOS Divas live in a place of abundance (being your authentic self, making choices that make you happy, being grateful), not a place of lack (comparing yourself to everyone else, trying to be someone you are not, striving for perfection).

Mind Your Business

Living mindfully is a key element of living like a PCOS Diva. People who live mindfully are aware of the day minute by minute and appreciate the present moment's abundance and challenges. In a world where no one seems to pay complete attention to anything, mindfulness is a powerful tool to help you avoid being overwhelmed.

Living mindfully helps PCOS Divas stay calm and centered. From this place, we can make good choices and keep the bigger picture in mind. For example, before my kids come home and the afternoon chaos begins, I make time for my afternoon snack and cup of tea. I do my best to sit for a few moments and savor it. I don't check my email while I snack. I don't fold laundry. I sit and enjoy a few minutes with my food. I think about what I am eating and simply experience the quiet moment. It isn't always easy to carve out these few minutes, but I do my best to do it each day.

For most of us, it's impossible to live mindfully all the time. Rather, it's an ebb and flow. You are mindful, you lose your focus, and then you are mindful again. Repeat. The constant ebb and flow helps us appreciate the practice. There are three keys to mindfulness:

1. **The past is the past.** We can waste a lot of time thinking about the past and what might have been. "What if I had been diagnosed earlier?" "What if I recognized the signs?" PCOS Divas don't waste their time rehashing the past. We think about the present and the future and move forward. Starting today, think about the person you strive to be and let today's decisions be the decisions that your "ideal PCOS Diva self" would make.

2. **Be in the present and grateful for today.** Every day is a gift. Every day you are given is another day full of possibilities and choices. Make the most of it! Appreciate the little blessings that happen and learn to appreciate the challenges. Together, they make your journey. Remember that the happiest people aren't necessarily those who are dealt the best hands; rather, they are those who make the best of the cards they're dealt. During the Healing PCOS 21-Day Plan, you will spend a few moments each day with gratitude. You may be surprised how even these few moments will change your life.

3. **Don't fear the future.** It is important to have long-term goals and look forward in order to anticipate roadblocks. That said, don't let the vastness and complete unpredictability of the future overwhelm you. Your life is full of fantastic possibilities, and the road to get there is long and winding. Don't lose the experience of the journey in a rush to get to your destination. Instead, try to live mindfully and manage your life moment to moment. For instance, when you are diagnosed with PCOS, you are initially overwhelmed with questions like, "Will I ever get pregnant?" and "Will I get diabetes?" Instead of zipping straight to these unanswerable questions, be mindful of the moment and get yourself on the path to wellness. Instead, ask, "What can I do today to start healing my body?" The steps you take to manage the issues of the day (insulin resistance, stress, etc.) will put you on the right track for the issues of the future (fertility, health).

———————— "No" Is a Complete Sentence ————————

In order to be mindful, we need to set priorities. You cannot be "in the moment" if you have to be in three places during that moment. For many of us, saying no can be difficult. We are programmed to accommodate as many people as possible, especially if they are important to us. In fact, you likely spend more time doing things for other people than you do for yourself.

Saying no and making yourself a priority does not have to be impolite or harsh. It isn't selfish. You are simply setting priorities that help you do what you choose to do well and completely. In this age of multitasking, very little is ever truly done as well as it could be. We are pushed to the edge of our capacity.

Instead of feeling as though you have to justify it to yourself when to say no, try justifying what you say yes to. Say yes to the things that make you happy, give you enjoyment, benefit you, contribute positively to your health, or add meaning to your life. Setting boundaries enables us to live mindfully. Not only is this empowering; it's necessary to your well-being and the well-being of those around you.

"When we stop listening to that voice in our head telling us we are not enough, we discover a voice in our soul who knows with certainty that we are more than enough."

—CRYSTAL ANDRUS MORISSETTE

The Most Important Piece

If you have ever taken a commercial flight, you have heard the speech the flight attendant gives about oxygen masks. It goes something like this: *"In the event of decompression, an oxygen mask will appear in front of you. To start the flow of oxygen, pull the mask toward you, place it firmly over your nose and mouth, and breathe normally. If you are traveling with a child or someone requiring assistance, secure your mask first; then assist the other person."*

Thinking like a PCOS Diva works much the same way. In order to thrive and be of service to those around you, you must first love and take care of yourself (or put on your oxygen mask). You are no good to anyone if you can't breathe.

Taking care of yourself is not selfish. It is necessary.

The key to thinking like a PCOS Diva is knowing that you *deserve* to feel good. Again, this is the critical mindset shift that will keep you on the path to thriving with PCOS. You must love yourself and recognize that you are worth the time, effort, and expense of being healthy and happy.

When you feel this self-worth, put effort into self-care, and really invest in self-love, the pieces will come together. You will feel better, and when you do, you will radiate this love to others. Your capacity to do good and be of help increases exponentially.

No, this does not mean you become an obnoxious diva, only worried about herself. You will not be demanding only green M&Ms in your dressing room. Holiday dinners with the family do not need to completely conform to your dietary choices. Self-love manifests itself in self-care. It means that you will respect yourself and your health enough to make time to care for yourself (mentally and physically), make self-respectful choices about what to eat and how to fit movement into your day, and speak to yourself in an encouraging and positive manner.

"Rest and self-care are so important. When you take time to replenish your spirit, it allows you to serve others from the overflow. You cannot serve from an empty vessel."

—ELEANOR BROWNN

Six Ways You Can Practice Self-Care

1. **Eat like a PCOS Diva.** In the next chapter, we will discuss how to eat like a PCOS Diva. You will learn new habits that reach way beyond *what* to eat. You will learn *how* to plan meals and grocery shop, avoid pitfalls and weather cravings, and read your body's signals and *where* to invest time and money in choosing the right foods to nourish your beautiful body.

2. **Move like a PCOS Diva.** In Chapter 5, we will explore ways to take self-care in a new direction: movement. You will find ways to move that you enjoy and look forward to doing. Stress relief, symptom relief, and joy will be the products of your work in this chapter.

3. **Reduce stress.** We have already spoken a little about stress. You know that stress releases the hormone cortisol, which wreaks havoc on your other hormones, immune system, and thyroid. Throughout the 21-Day Plan, we will practice stress relief as a critical part of self-care. You will learn how movement can reduce your stress levels. You will learn to meditate in order to center yourself and prepare for the stresses that you encounter every day. You will practice mindfulness and learn to savor seemingly mundane moments (and even stressful ones). Finally, you will learn to diffuse stressful situations with on-the-spot stress relief.

4. **Get adequate sleep.** We don't need research to tell us that sleep is critical for brain function, but there's plenty of it out there. We've all experienced the groggy feeling, poor decision making, and memory loss after a night of little or no sleep. Did you know that studies also show the clear relationship between sleep, food consumption, weight regulation, and metabolism? Chronic sleep deprivation impacts every system and hormone in your body. Your body's ability to signal when to eat, process glucose, and repair cells are all affected. As a result, you become forgetful, can't process insulin and glucose properly, have increased inflammation, make bad food choices, and gain weight. There are countless reasons for this sleep deprivation, including cortisol

or melatonin imbalances, medications, medical conditions, and lack of self-care. In the 21-Day Plan, you will learn sleep habits that will (most nights) help you get the rest you desperately need.

5. **Find a creative outlet.** Using your creativity is healing, whether you write, dance, scrapbook, draw, paint, quilt, sing, play an instrument, or color (I love adult coloring books). Any sort of artistic expression can stimulate stress relief and help you express yourself. Throughout the 21-Day Plan, you'll make time to tap into your creative side as part of your self-care regimen.

6. **Indulge.** Being a PCOS Diva isn't about deprivation and denial. That is no way to live. Being a PCOS Diva is about living your best life and taking steps to make that possible. An important part of that is taking time for yourself, even just a few minutes per day, and replacing old destructive habits with joyous, indulgent, positive ones. Think about how you reward yourself or relax. Do you grab a pint of Ben & Jerry's? Sack out on the couch with movies for the afternoon? It might feel good to do those things in the moment, but afterward you are left feeling lousy. Consider replacing these habits with others that make you feel great long term. In the 21-Day Plan, you will begin your very own "Sweet Stuff" list of things you can do to indulge a little. We all need them.

Starting Today

You will start thinking like a PCOS Diva. You will stop being a victim and partner with your body. You will do your best to be patient with yourself, acknowledge that you deserve to feel great, and take the steps to be that way. You will begin and end your days with gratitude for all you have and the beauty around you.

These invisible changes will soon have very visible results that benefit both you and the people around you. You are not being selfish when practicing self-care. You are investing in yourself in order to reap rewards for your friends, family, and coworkers. They will notice the difference. But what's more important is that *you* will.

4

Eat like a PCOS Diva

I was raised in the 1980s and 1990s, the era of margarine, diet soda, and fat-free everything. As a teen, I wouldn't have been caught dead with a package of Oreos, but a fistful of fat-free Snackwells cookies sounded like a good choice. Wash them down with some Diet Coke, and I had a good "skinny" snack. Looking back, it is no wonder I felt terrible. Not only was I not getting the nutrients I needed, but I was filling my body with artificial chemicals and inflammatory foods that wreaked havoc on my hormones.

The pattern continued into college. My body was crying out for protein, and I was answering the cry by secretly binging on peanut butter. I should take this moment to apologize to my old college roommates. I admit it. I was the Peanut Butter Bandit. All those jars of peanut butter that went missing—that was me and my PCOS. I'm sorry. I didn't understand what my cravings were trying to tell me, and your stores of peanut butter paid the price.

To make matters worse, being a vegetarian was trendy and sounded like a healthy option, so I jumped on the bandwagon. Unfortunately, I wasn't a particularly good vegetarian. I ate almost no protein. Tofu sounded weird, and beans were not glamorous. I filled in the space where lean protein should have been with carbs.

Later in college, when I no longer had to eat in the cafeteria, I gave up vegetarianism and discovered both that I actually liked to cook and that I was pretty good at it. I began hosting dinner parties and cooking for myself and friends on a regular basis. I didn't put it together until much later, but I started feeling better. I was finally giving my body what it craved—lean, clean meats and vegetables!

A Healthy Relationship with Food

Let's talk about the second most important part of the PCOS Diva lifestyle: food. Many (dare I say most) women with PCOS have an adversarial relationship with food. In fact, a startling number of us have some level of eating disorder. Whether it is occasional binge eating, bulimia, or anorexia, our dysfunctional relationship with food may come from any number of sources, including:

- Struggling to conform with societal expectations for the perfect body.
- Unhealthy foods available to us in our youth that became our go-to or comfort foods.
- Emotional eating.
- Biological issues, such as chemical imbalances in the areas of the brain that regulate appetite, digestion, and hunger.
- Psychological issues, such as low self-esteem, feelings of inadequacy or lack of control in life, depression, anxiety, anger, stress, or loneliness.
- Interpersonal issues, such as troubled personal relationships, difficulty expressing emotions and feelings, a history of being teased or ridiculed based on size or weight, or a history of physical or sexual abuse.

PCOS Divas must approach their diet using the proper mindset. PCOS Divas do not engage in the three Ds: *deprivation*, *denial*, and *diet*. We feed ourselves (including our cravings) mindfully and with care. Our diet isn't a fad diet. It isn't restrictive, extreme, or punishing. It is a way of eating that springs from the PCOS Diva mindset. We eat foods that our bodies *deserve*, that make us feel strong, healthy, and energized. We are aware of how different foods make us feel, and we make

"Three years ago, I tried the 'next thing' after years of diets, medicines, and exercise programs. My 'next thing' was the PCOS Diva Jumpstart week. I never looked back. Feeling stronger and more in control of my choices, my body, and my PCOS, I began eating like a PCOS Diva all the time. So did my family. I lost thirty pounds in the first three months of living the PCOS Diva lifestyle. My three sons started requesting specific recipes and began reading labels on food products. Amy's research and information have transformed my life, my mood, and my family's dinner table. Her holistic approach is both achievable and down to earth, addressing habits, emotions, and roadblocks. Hundreds of tasty recipes, pages of tips to make and change habits, and prepared shopping lists equipped me for success."

—HEATHER G.

mindful choices accordingly. Our PCOS Diva mindset means that we nurture ourselves, and having a healthy relationship with food and choosing foods that heal, nourish, and taste delicious are an important part of that. During the Healing PCOS 21-Day Plan, you will develop a healthier relationship with food. It will become an enjoyable part of your daily self-care.

Treat Food as Medicine

Many diet books tell you to look at food as fuel for your body. Although this is true, food is much, much more than fuel. It doesn't just give us energy. The food we eat has the power to heal or harm us. It can make us feel energized and focused or sleepy, bloated, and constipated. We need to consider food medicine. The right foods can regulate insulin, control inflammation, regulate cardiovascular health, improve gut health, and help manage stress and PCOS symptoms. The nutrients, phytonutrients, antioxidants, fiber, vitamins, and minerals contained in the foods you choose can be the difference between healing diseases and disorders and making them worse. In fact, nutrigenomics is an entire field of research exploring the link between the food we take in and how those nutrients communicate with our genes to trigger or reduce the risk of certain diseases such as heart disease and diabetes. These interactions may even play a part in your cravings, fitness, and overall health.

Eating like a PCOS Diva means embracing a plant-based diet that includes healing foods: wild-caught fish, organic poultry, grass-fed meat, gluten-free whole grains, healthy fats, and tons of produce. You'll move out of the processed food aisles of your grocery store and into the produce section, where you'll discover fruits and vegetables that are low on the glycemic index, which means they will blow your mind and heal your body without spiking your blood sugar. No, you will not be eating crazy, exotic foods you have never heard of. That's not sustainable. But you may encounter new foods and learn new ways to prepare and appreciate some you already know. You will learn how different foods can work as medicine and help soothe your symptoms. For example:

Apples: Apples are low on the glycemic index and high in vitamin C, potassium, antioxidants, and fiber. Studies demonstrate that adding apples to your diet can reduce your risk of diabetes and weight gain.

Avocados: Avocados are packed with vitamins, minerals, and heart-healthy fatty acids that help quell systemic inflammation, promote healthy endocrine and immune system function, and make your skin glow. Adding an avocado per day to an already well-balanced diet has been shown to lower risk of heart disease, lower LDL cholesterol, and reduce oxidative stress.

Berries: Berries are packed with immune-boosting, cancer-preventing, heart-protecting, obesity-preventing antioxidant components, including specific polyphenols, flavonoids, and other phytocomponents that fight inflammation and disease. Researchers are learning that phytonutrients in raspberries may prevent obesity and fatty liver by regulating certain enzymes.

Brown rice: Unlike its nutritionally stripped white cousin, brown rice is a gluten-free whole grain containing vitamins, minerals, fiber, and protein to balance its carbs. Brown rice contains magnesium and selenium for heart health and manganese for bone and thyroid health, regulation of blood sugar levels, metabolism of fats and carbohydrates, and absorption of calcium. Fiber lowers blood glucose (and, as a result, insulin) and estrogen levels, all while flushing toxins.

Cinnamon: Rich in antioxidants, cinnamon can help stabilize blood sugar and reduce insulin resistance. Some studies indicate that it may also help regulate menstruation.

Dark chocolate: Chocolate containing 70 percent cacao or more reduces hypertension, increases circulation, aids in preventing atherosclerosis, improves glucose regulation by preventing blood sugar spikes, and may promote weight loss by controlling hunger and promoting satiety. It can also improve mood, soothe nerves, prevent memory decline, and improve overall cognitive function. As an added bonus, it contains all-important magnesium, which can help regulate insulin, relieve anxiety, boost energy, and support bone health.

Green tea: A zero-calorie beverage, green tea is considered one of the world's healthiest drinks. Green tea contains a high concentration of powerful antioxidants that improve blood flow, lower cholesterol, improve hypertension, and may prevent other heart-related issues, including congestive heart failure and stroke. Because of its circulatory benefits, green tea also nourishes and stimulates the brain by boosting brain activity and memory and helps block the formation of amyloid plaques linked to Alzheimer's disease.

Leafy greens: Romaine and red leaf lettuce, kale, chard, spinach, collards, beet greens, dandelion greens, endive, basil, parsley, and arugula are the very best low-calorie, high-fiber, low–glycemic index food sources of essential vitamins and minerals. They improve digestion, absorption of nutrients in the gut, glucose regulation, and overall endocrine function and reduce the risk of metabolic, cardiovascular, and autoimmune diseases, as well as cancer. Leafy greens are also a good source of many B vitamins, especially folate.

Maple syrup: With fewer calories than honey and a lower glycemic index than cane sugar, maple syrup is a great natural sweetener choice. It contains water, protein, fat, carbohydrates, antioxidants, calcium, iron, magnesium, phosphorus sodium, potassium, zinc, thiamin, riboflavin, manganese, niacin, and B_6.

Nuts and seeds: Eating nuts and seeds in combination with fruit or other high–glycemic index foods lowers the total glycemic index and improves glucose and insulin regulation. Seeds (especially pumpkin seeds, sesame seeds, and cashews) contain essential fatty acids (EFAs) and zinc, which our bodies need. EFAs help regulate hormone function; improve hair, skin, and nails; lower insulin levels; stabilize blood sugars; and help regulate periods. These may also help with hirsutism.

Oats: Both rolled and steel-cut oats are nutritional powerhouses, though steel-cut oats are lower on the glycemic index. These gluten-free whole grains contain fiber, protein, antioxidants, and tons of vitamins and minerals, including manganese, phosphorous, magnesium, copper, iron, zinc, B_1, B_5, and folate. Thanks to the high fiber content, oats keep you feeling full while helping to lower your blood sugar and improve insulin sensitivity.

Buying Organic

When choosing meat, poultry, fish, fats like butter, fruits, and vegetables, consider organic, grass-fed, and wild-caught options. These are likely to contain fewer of the toxins that creep into conventional foods through pesticides, antibiotics, water, and feed. Some fruits and vegetables are especially prone to contamination; others are more resistant. The Environmental Working Group (ewg.org) keeps list of the "Dirty Dozen" and "Clean Fifteen" as well as a seafood guide on its website.

Listen to Your Body

Partnering with your body and listening to its signals will provide you with a wealth of valuable information on your healing journey. During the 21-Day Plan, you'll learn:

To identify the foods that heal and those that hurt you. Do you need a nap an hour after eating a salad? What if you add chicken or a healthy fat like avocado or olive oil? Does adding croutons make you crave more carbs and feel logy later? For the next few weeks, you will use a journal to log *what* you eat and how you *feel* after you eat it. How do you feel an hour after your morning smoothie? Energized? Hungry? How do you feel after snacking on crackers and cheese? Bloated? Grouchy? Some effects can be felt in the short term while others may not present until hours later. Keeping a food journal will help you to spot the patterns and develop a personalized eating plan that nurtures *your* body. When you stop listening to fad diets and their one-size-fits-all promises and start listening to your body, you will be surprised by what you hear.

To recognize what your body needs. Cravings are your body's way of telling you it needs something. No, it is not telling you that it needs some chocolate ice cream. Are you craving chocolate? You may need magnesium. Are you craving salty snacks? Your diet may be missing certain minerals such as calcium or magnesium. Are you craving sweets? Your blood sugar may be low. Are you craving carbohydrates? Your hormones are probably fluctuating. Sometimes, you aren't really hungry at all; you may just be dehydrated. Is the craving emotional? Many of us eat reflexively when we are bored, sad, or tired. What we think is a craving is really just a habitual reaction to our state of mind, or we may use food to fill hungers in other areas of our lives.

Sometimes I just want a potato chip. There is something about the salt and crunch that my body craves. When I get this feeling, I ask myself what's going on. Maybe I need more minerals and crave the salt. Sometimes I find that I am frustrated, and crunching on something like chips helps me take out my frustration. Sometimes I find another way to do this, and sometimes I decide to mindfully indulge. The important thing is to recognize what drives your craving.

Sometimes when a craving strikes (especially for a food that I know makes me sick), I tell myself, "I can have this food anytime. This is not the last time I will ever see it. I choose not to eat it right now." This mindset helps me get some distance from the immediacy of the feeling.

Try to follow the 80/20 rule. Eat exactly what your body needs 80 percent of the time. The other 20 percent is for those times that you indulge, slip, or otherwise fall off the wagon. You will notice that, as you upgrade your everyday diet and start to crowd out processed foods, you will start to crave nourishing rather than unhealthy food.

--- ## Sugar-Craving Busters ---

Typically, we should listen to our body's cravings and try to supply the nutrients it is signaling for, but with sugar our craving is often an indication of an addiction. Until we break the addiction, feeding this craving is not helping. Here are four Sugar-Craving Busters that may help:

1. L-glutamine is an amino acid that has been found to reduce or even eliminate sugar and carb cravings. Try a 500 mg dose up to three times a day when sugar cravings occur. This dose should rid you of sugar cravings within a month or two.

2. Coconut manna (also called coconut butter) is pure coconut flesh blended until it reaches the consistency of peanut butter. Eat a spoonful of this healthy fat straight from the jar or spread it on a piece of dark chocolate when you are dying for something sweet.

3. Mineral deficiencies can cause cravings, so drink a glass of high-quality mineral water, like San Pellegrino, to replace the trace minerals you may be lacking. Try this especially if you regularly drink filtered water.

4. Drink licorice mint tea with a little coconut oil to curb cravings. I also like Good Earth Organic Sweet & Spicy Caffeine-Free Tea for sweet cravings at night.

During the next 21 days, we will talk more about what to do when you have a craving. Until then, don't fight your body. When you are craving something, first ask what your body may be telling you. Then try to give it what it needs. Remember, *nothing tastes as good as feeling good feels*.

Listening to your body takes practice. Be patient with yourself. By the end of the 21-Day Plan, you will be much more in tune with your body's signals.

Choose Foods That Heal the Root Cause of Your Symptoms

Anti-inflammatory Foods

Chronic inflammation is the root cause of many of your PCOS symptoms, such as insulin resistance and acne. Every time you consume a food to which you are allergic or sensitive, your body reacts as though it is under attack, and inflammation results. This inflammation is recognized by your adrenal glands as stress. With your body under attack, the adrenals go into overdrive producing cortisol to get you through the emergency. As a result, they produce less estrogen, progesterone, and testosterone, causing hormonal imbalance. If inflammation in your digestive tract is left unchecked, it can result in leaky gut syndrome, causing inflammation throughout your body and leading to a variety of autoimmune diseases.

Removing inflammatory foods from your diet is imperative. Determining which foods to eliminate from your diet is a process. Just as every woman with PCOS has a different set of symptoms, we each have different food allergies and sensitivities. A food allergy triggers an immune-system reaction, resulting in a range of symptoms such as hives, swelling, and trouble breathing. You may know almost right away if you have an allergy, but it could take four hours or more. A food sensitivity is an adverse reaction to a food that does not involve the immune system. Symptoms, including bloating, gas, diarrhea, nausea, and indigestion, may emerge hours or days after consumption.

The nine most common food allergens are:

1. Peanuts
2. Tree nuts
3. Milk
4. Eggs
5. Wheat and other grains containing gluten, including barley and rye
6. Soy
7. Fish
8. Shellfish
9. Corn

Over the next three weeks, you'll begin to pinpoint your food sensitivities. Your food journal will help you to identify the foods that make you feel miserable, and as part of the 21-Day Plan you will limit or eliminate three inflammatory foods that commonly affect women with PCOS: gluten, dairy, and processed soy.

Gluten: Many women with PCOS have a gluten sensitivity. For those with celiac disease, an autoimmune disorder, gluten must be avoided entirely. Most of us have a sensitivity that results in constant low-grade inflammation.

Gluten-free doesn't mean healthy. There are tons of gluten-free products available now. Many of them are terrific alternatives for foods that make us sick. However, a gluten-free cookie is still a cookie. It is loaded with sugar and other ingredients that are not good for you. "Gluten-free" on the label is not a free pass to consume junk.

Dairy: Most humans stop producing the enzymes needed to properly digest and metabolize milk (and foods containing milk, such as cheese and yogurt) after they have been weaned. In fact, much of the world's adult population may be unable to digest lactose, a sugar found in milk. Those who are lactose intolerant experience digestive issues whenever they consume dairy products.

Others may react poorly to the casein and whey proteins found in milk. According to Dr. Amy Myers, 50 percent of people who are gluten intolerant are also casein intolerant due to the similar molecular structures. In addition, your body may struggle to manage the acidity, hormones, and antibiotics that are often present. Grass-fed butter and ghee are allowed as they contain no or very minimal amounts of casein or lactose, and provide multiple health benefits.

Soy: Women with PCOS should limit their exposure to soy, not only because it is one of the most common allergens, but also because it interferes with hormones. Soybean protein naturally contains phytoestrogens called isoflavones that may mimic the activity of the hormone estrogen in your body. Soy is also a goitrogen, a substance that suppresses the thyroid gland and interferes with thyroid hormone production. If you must consume soy, please choose organic and/or fermented products in small amounts.

When *Not* to Eat: Intermittent Fasting

Intermittent fasting is a hot topic right now. The truth is, it is nothing new. Our ancestors went for long stretches between meals due to scarcity. Our bodies are designed to rest and digest between meals. Modern intermittent fasting refers to stretching out the time between your evening and morning meal or greatly reducing the amount of food you consume a couple of days each week. Research tells us that intermittent fasting can help cellular regeneration, lower insulin levels, boost weight loss, and fight stress and inflammation as well as reduce depression and improve brain health.

Intermittent fasting isn't for everyone. If you have an eating disorder, diabetes, or an impaired metabolism, skipping meals may be more than your body can handle. Finally, if you notice dizziness or you stop getting your period, stop fasting.

I suggest trying to fast four days a week. On these days, create a twelve-hour gap between dinner and breakfast (for example, 6 p.m. to 6 a.m.) in which you don't eat at all. Experiment and see if this works for you.

Eliminating these three allergens during the 21-Day Plan will reduce inflammation and help you determine if you are sensitive to gluten, dairy, and/or soy. Later, you may want to try reintroducing them into your diet one at a time and watching closely for signs of trouble. Experience tells me that you'll notice a difference right away.

I use tree nuts, fish, and eggs in many PCOS Diva recipes because they offer fantastic health benefits. Please skip those if you know you are sensitive to them! If you're feeling better after eliminating milk, gluten, and soy, consider removing the other common allergens one at a time and paying attention to your body's response in order to identify other inflammatory foods you should avoid.

Foods That Balance Your Blood Sugar Level

Sugar and carbohydrates can throw your insulin off balance, setting off a cascade of cravings, fatigue, moodiness, and hormonal imbalance. Avoid processed foods and experiment with low–glycemic index carbohydrate choices, such as berries.

--------- Symptoms of Falling Blood Sugar ---------

- Sweating (especially at the back of the neck below the hairline)

- Nervousness, shakiness, and weakness

- Extreme hunger and slight nausea

- Headache

- Fast heartbeat

- Irritability and mood swings

- Sleep disturbances (night sweats, confusion upon waking, nightmares, waking suddenly)

- Dizziness

- Blurred vision

- Anxiety

If you have trouble recognizing how different foods affect your blood sugar, try using a glucometer, a tool that measures the approximate amount of glucose in your blood. When I began experimenting with my diet, I realized that I had become totally disconnected from my body's blood-sugar signals. I didn't connect the pizza I ate to the energy crash two hours later. The glucometer helped me connect the dots. Though not required, I encourage you to give a glucometer a try, adjust your food choices, and talk to your doctor about your findings next time you visit.

The PCOS Diva Plate

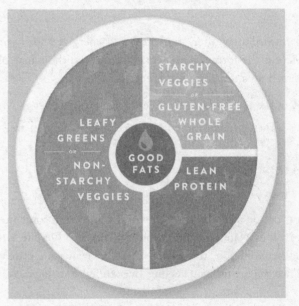

Two of the biggest challenges fledgling PCOS Divas face are discerning serving sizes and eating the right combination of protein, carbs, and fats at each meal. The PCOS Diva Plate will help you quickly determine how much to eat of each food and eliminate calorie and carb counting. That can take the pleasure out of a nice meal fast.

Every PCOS Diva is unique, so experiment with your combinations. You will know you have the right combination when you feel

Fat Is Your Friend

Well, some fats are your friend. Among the many benefits, good fats aid
nutrient absorption and improve satiety. Try these healthy fats:

- Avocado and avocado oil
- Grass-fed butter
- Extra-virgin olive oil
- Virgin coconut oil, coconut manna
- Nuts and seeds and butters made from them
- Fish and fish oil

---

satisfied immediately after your meal and energized for hours afterward. Here is the formula that works for me and thousands of PCOS
Divas. Based on a medium-size dinner plate:

Fill ½ of the plate with leafy greens or nonstarchy veggies.

Fill ¼ of the plate with starchy root veggies *or* a gluten-free whole
grain.

Fill ¼ of the plate with a lean protein.

Add a generous portion of healthy fat.

As you eat, be mindful about how full you feel. At some meals, you
may clear your plate; at others, you will eat less. Despite what your
grandmother told you, there is no need to clean your plate at every
meal. That may leave you feeling overstuffed and logy. What's the
point?

If you choose to have seconds, keep the PCOS Diva Plate in mind.
If you take more grains, have more protein and veggies in proportion.

Eating on the Go

You've heard the old adage, "Breakfast is the most important meal of
the day." At least, that's what cereal companies want us to think. For
women with PCOS, though, breakfast really *is* critical. A solid break-

fast can help to keep our blood-sugar levels even. Please don't skip it because you are running out the door or feel nauseous when you wake up. This nausea may be attributed to low blood sugar and eating will usually help.

During the next 21 days, you will experiment with the kind of breakfast that works best for you. You will find a few favorites and establish a routine that basically automates breakfast. Try to incorporate some protein and greens every morning. I do this by having a protein smoothie almost every day. I can take it with me in the car, and it will give me sure-fire energy until lunch. Steel-cut oats travel well too. Make some protein bars, and eat one in the car if you must. The point is to find something that nourishes you first thing and keeps you fueled throughout your morning.

Lunch is our chance to refuel, and PCOS Divas have a secret to the perfect lunch—automation. I have two tricks to help you accomplish this. First, as you clean up dinner, package up the right PCOS Diva Plate combination of leftovers for your lunch tomorrow. Your coworkers will

Tips for Dining Out

- Use www.findmeglutenfree.com or the app to help identify restaurants.

- Visit a restaurant's menu online before you go, so you can plan what you'll order.

- If all else fails, request grilled or broiled chicken or fish and then ask for whatever fresh veggies they have in the kitchen.

- Have the bread basket taken away, so you're not tempted (even if it is gluten-free).

- Choose dishes that have a lot of veggies and some lean protein, and ask if the veggies can be lightly sautéed or steamed.

- Ask the server to bring you some olive oil or real butter and fresh lemon to flavor the veggies.

- Request a double serving of vegetables to replace the white potatoes or rice that often accompanies dinner.

- Order sparkling water with a squeeze of lime or lemon.

envy your gorgeous lunches, and it will save you time in the morning. Second, salad in a jar can be made days ahead. Just grab and go!

Snacks work much the same way. We will plan snacks ahead of time, so that you have them on hand when you need one. Try to keep emergency snacks stashed in convenient places, like your purse, car, or desk. No more trips to the vending machine for you!

Every PCOS Diva deserves a night off. Once in a while, go out to a restaurant and let someone else cook for a change. It is also a chance to strengthen your PCOS Diva muscles. Remember my story at the beginning of this book about ordering a sweet potato? Many restaurants now have gluten-free and/or healthy options already on their menus. If they don't, just ask! Trust me, you will not be the first person to ever ask them to "hold the bun" or whether there is dairy in a sauce. It's not rude to ask. They want you to be a satisfied customer as much as you want to feel good. If you find that isn't true, find a different restaurant next time. Be a PCOS Diva! You deserve to eat well and feel great.

Can I Be a PCOS Diva
and a Vegetarian/Vegan?

In my experience working with women with PCOS, it is difficult to manage PCOS on a vegetarian/vegan diet. Women often trade animal protein for processed soy (which throws hormones off balance) and large quantities of beans (which can spike blood sugar). That doesn't mean you can't have meatless meals during the week; it's just difficult to be completely exclusive without intensive help from a nutrition professional.

Drink like a PCOS Diva

Americans each consume roughly 66 pounds of added sugar per year. That's about 20 teaspoons per day! Much of that comes from our beverages. Sodas and other soft drinks like lemonade and iced tea are the main culprits. Also, watch your coffee. You might be shocked to know how much sugar is in the latte from your favorite coffee shop. As PCOS Divas, we don't drink our calories. Diet-soda lovers, don't think you are off the hook either (see below).

The problem isn't just the extra calories. The sugar in these drinks kicks off the unhealthy insulin cycle that we are working so hard to get under control. These sugary and often caffeinated beverages can also overstimulate the adrenals as well as cause anxiety and oxidative stress. Upgrading your daily beverages may mean changing a very ingrained habit, but if you are mindful about your choices, it will soon become second nature.

PCOS Diva Beverages

PCOS Divas drink:

Warm water with lemon in the morning. Lemon water is a great way to hydrate and energize first thing. It also will reduce bloating and help you better absorb nutrients all day.

Infused water. Experts say we need 64 ounces of water every day. I find that women with PCOS need more. Make 64 ounces your minimum and adjust up from there. Jazz it up and make it even better for you with these add-ins, but don't feel limited to these. Get creative! Just try to use low–glycemic index fruits.

- Lemon stimulates the liver and helps release digestive enzymes. Lemon water contains useful antioxidants and electrolytes (potassium, calcium, and magnesium) and is a rich source of the immune-boosting vitamin C.
- Ginger is a great pain reliever for many things from menstrual cramps to headaches. It's also energizing and smells fabulous. Make a pitcher of ginger tea to drink throughout the day. Grate a 1- to 2-inch piece of ginger root. Add 3 to 4 cups of water and a squeeze of lemon. Strain and serve over ice.
- Strawberries are packed with vitamins, minerals, and other antioxidants. They contain potassium, vitamin K, and

magnesium, which are important for bone health, and biotin, which is good for your hair and nails. They also can help ease inflammation.

- Coconut water contains antioxidants, amino acids, enzymes, and minerals like iron, calcium, potassium, magnesium, manganese, and zinc as well as vitamin C and B vitamins. Add a splash!
- Herbs, such as mint, lavender, or basil, can be refreshing.

Mineral water or seltzer. Bubbly beverages like mineral water and seltzer are great replacements for soda. Add a splash of fruit juice or real fruit for added flavor.

Tea. Studies have shown that green and spearmint teas can reduce androgens, but there are health benefits in all teas (see box on p. 69). If you need a sweetener, try a little stevia or honey.

Apple cider vinegar. Full of enzymes, good bacteria, and acetic acid, apple cider vinegar has been shown to drop blood sugar levels by 6 percent. Studies have shown it works as effectively as metformin in people with insulin resistance. Drink the following beverage before each meal to improve insulin sensitivity and prevent blood-sugar spikes:

To a 12- to 16-ounce glass of water add:

  2 teaspoons apple cider vinegar

  2 teaspoons lemon juice (balances blood sugar levels and contains vitamin C)

  A sprinkle of ground cinnamon (a fat-soluble antioxidant that lowers blood sugar)

  A dash of cayenne pepper (optional; can reduce blood sugar)

If you are on metformin, consult your doctor. Combining apple cider vinegar and metformin may make your blood sugar too low.

PCOS Divas Don't Drink Diet Soda

During my Discover Your PCOS Diva Jumpstart Program, I ask participants to eliminate soda, especially diet soda. Since many women switched to diet soda from regular soda to save calories, they are shocked to find that the swap does them no good. It may even make things worse. And now they're addicted. So why is diet soda a big PCOS Diva no-no?

It confuses your body. The artificial sweetener in diet soda is so sweet that it dulls your senses over time, so you will eventually not recognize when you are consuming sugary things. The result is that you consume sweeter and sweeter things to get the same sensation; natural sugars in fruit will no longer sate your sugar craving. In addition, according to the Harvard School of Public Health, "By providing a sweet taste without any calories . . . artificial sweeteners cause us to crave more sweet foods and drinks, which can add up to excess calories."

It raises your risk of diabetes, stroke, and heart disease. A recent study shows that people who drink diet soda every day increase their risk of metabolic syndrome (high blood pressure, abnormal cholesterol levels, excess body fat around the waist) by 36 percent, which raises the risk of diabetes, stroke, and heart disease.

It doesn't help you lose weight. Typically, people who drink diet soda make up for the calories they "saved" somewhere else. I'm sure you've seen people order a Big Mac with a Diet Coke. In fact, many studies show that diet-soda drinkers have a larger waist circumference than those who do not drink diet soda. People who consume two or more diet sodas per day have an even greater increase in weight around the middle—what researchers called "a striking dose-response relationship."

It is associated with depression. Studies show that people who consume four or more cans of soda per day (diet or otherwise) are 30 percent more likely to develop depression than those who do not consume sugary drinks.

It increases your risk of osteoporosis. Tufts University researchers found that female cola (caffeinated or decaffeinated) drinkers had lower bone mineral density in their hips than women who didn't drink soda regardless of age, body mass index, physical activity, alcohol intake, and other factors. Again, frequency of consumption matters. "Women who drink cola daily had lower bone mineral density than those who drink it only once a week," explains lead researcher Katherine Tucker.

It has no nutritional value. Other than a small amount of water, soda is made entirely of artificial ingredients that, at best, offer no nourishment.

Phasing out diet soda is an act of self-care. I understand the deep psychological attachment and know that it can be a hard habit to break. Start small. First, decide that you want to stop. Then slowly begin upgrading to healthier beverages until diet sodas are crowded out and your taste buds return to normal.

PCOS Divas Sometimes Drink Wine

One of the world's favorite indulgences is wine. Many of my clients like a glass at the end of the day to help unwind. That's totally fine. If you are a wine lover, I encourage you to savor a glass of red wine with a meal, but no more than three times a week. Why so infrequently?

Wine weakens resolve. You are much more likely to make PCOS-unfriendly choices if you have more than a glass.

Wine depresses the function of your adrenal glands. Inadequately functioning adrenals can lead to issues with inflammation and sleep patterns.

That said, there are health benefits to wine. It is widely understood that, in moderation, wine can support cardiovascular health. We now know that red wine (pinot noir especially) contains resveratrol, which has noted anti-inflammatory, antioxidant, anti-aging, and cardioprotective properties. In addition, new research indicates that resveratrol may "help moderate the hormone imbalance that is one of the central features of PCOS." Unfortunately, in order to metabolize enough resveratrol to make an impact, supplementation is needed. It is not feasible or safe to drink that much wine.

So go ahead and indulge in a glass of wine, but be sure to enjoy it with a meal to lesson your blood-sugar response.

Tea

Tea is an important part of my self-care. The ritual of preparing tea is calming, and the unique flavor of each infusion is one of my "sweet treats." Beyond these benefits, tea can be used medicinally by women with PCOS to help with some of the toughest and most common symptoms.

Insulin resistance. Studies show that regular consumption of tea can reduce insulin resistance, a precursor of diabetes and weight gain. Black, green, ginger, turmeric, and cinnamon tea are all effective.

Androgen excess. Tea's anti-androgenic effects and ability to modulate estrogen production make it a popular treatment for PCOS. Spearmint, red reishi, licorice, Chinese peony, and green teas all have androgen-lowering effects.

Mood, stress, and anxiety. Tea is an excellent stress reliever. Tea contains an amino acid called L-theanine, which studies show creates a state of deep relaxation and mental alertness. In addition, researchers have found that tea promotes a sense of calm distinct from its chemical impact on our body and brain. In this way, drinking tea is an act of self-care. I especially like matcha and chamomile teas when I'm stressed.

Inflammation. Tea has been used for centuries to fight inflammation, and modern science has finally verified its analgesic and anti-inflammatory properties, particularly in green tea varieties. This means relief for PCOS symptoms such as acne, headaches, and fatigue, and it may lessen weight gain and decrease your risk of diabetes.

Use Supplements to Fill in Gaps

There is no "perfect" diet. Even a well-balanced diet will have nutritional gaps. Women with PCOS often benefit from herbal supplements to help with specific symptoms such as insulin resistance, inflammation, hormone balance, or stress.

So why can't we simply upgrade our diets and get the nutrients we need? The following are the main reasons women with PCOS may find themselves to be nutrient deficient.

Deficient diet. The Standard American Diet (SAD)—a diet high in sugar and refined carbohydrates and low in lean meats and vegetables—seems an obvious reason for nutrient deficiency. Many Americans are overfed and undernourished as a result of SAD. For women with PCOS, this diet induces high levels of insulin, which stimulate androgen receptors on the ovaries and cause many of the most common symptoms, such as hirsutism, thin hair on the head, and acne. Our bodies signal this lack of nutrients with increasing intensity as the problem goes on. Eventually, diabetes may develop. Studies specifically find that zinc, magnesium, chromium, and vitamin D are commonly deficient in patients with diabetes and women with PCOS.

Even if you have upgraded your diet to include lots of vegetables and lean meats, the foods available to the general public no longer contain the high levels of nutrients they enjoyed historically. Modern agricultural methods have stripped nutrients from the soil. The blueberries you eat today probably do not contain the same amount of nutrients that blueberries did when your grandmother ate them.

Nutrient conversion issues. Research demonstrates that many women with PCOS are unable to convert vitamins and minerals into the forms needed in the body.

Methylenetetrahydrofolate reductase (MTHFR). This gene instructs the body to make an enzyme that converts folic acid (B_9) into a useable form, folate. When this occurs, we say it has been methylated. If you have the MTHFR mutation, your body is less efficient at making the conversion and therefore utilizing the folic acid in multivitamins and prenatal vitamins, which is important in preventing serious birth defects. A lack of folate may also result in lethargy, mood disorders, and impaired cognitive function. MTHFR is also responsible for converting homocysteine into methionine, which you need for growth, cell repair, and metabolism. High levels of homocysteine in the blood may negatively affect mood and mental health and are associated with cardiovascular disease, high blood pressure, depression, migraines, and more. A high-quality supplement containing folate instead of folic acid can help. I suggest all women with PCOS be tested for the MTHFR mutation.

Delta-6-desaturase (D6D). Foods such as flaxseed, leafy greens, and walnuts are high in an omega-3 fatty acid called alpha-linolenic acid (ALA). Omega 3s are widely recommended for their many health benefits, especially for the brain, eyes, and heart. For women with PCOS, sufficient amounts of omega 3s can improve fertility, regulate hormones, improve insulin sensitivity, stave off inflammation, reduce hirsutism, and reduce the risk of fatty liver and heart disease. Unfortunately, for ALA to be used in the body, it must first be converted by an enzyme called delta-6-desaturase (D6D) into one of two other omega-3 fatty acids, docosahexaenoic acid (DHA) or eicosapentaenoic acid (EPA). This transformation is very inefficient and is further inhibited by elevated cholesterol, caffeine or alcohol consumption, saturated fat or trans-fat consumption, vitamin and mineral deficiencies, and hormonal abnormalities, insulin resistance, and hypothyroidism. Even when D6D functions normally, only about 8 to 20 percent of ALA is converted to EPA and 0.5 to 9 percent to DHA (this may be slightly higher in women of childbearing age or who are pregnant). The omega 3s found in fish (and fish oil) are already in the form of DHA and EPA, so they do not need to undergo this conversion and are more bioavailable. Still, it is hard to safely eat enough fish to meet the daily requirements.

Inositol. Inositol is a vitamin found in whole-grain foods and made by your body from glucose. *Myo-inositol* and *D-chiro-inositol* are two of the nine naturally occurring inositols that people need. These two inositols help with insulin sensitization, and women with PCOS commonly benefit from supplementation.

Found in meat, myo-inositol is critical for properly functioning insulin receptors. It has also been linked to the activation of serotonin (a "feel good" hormone) receptors, which could relieve depression and improve appetite, mood, and anxiety. Supplementation may help with inducing menses and ovulation and reducing acne and hirsutism. Myo-inositol is found in food, but women with PCOS often have a defect in their insulin pathways, which are heavily reliant on inositols. Adding myo-inositol supplementation seems to alleviate the problem.

Not abundant in our diets, D-chiro-inositol (DCI) needs to be converted from other inositols (myo-inositol and D-pinitol) by the body in order to be used. Studies suggest that women with PCOS may not be able to efficiently convert other inositols to DCI. Low levels of DCI have commonly been observed in women with impaired insulin sensitivity and PCOS. DCI increases the action of insulin, improves ovulatory function, and decreases serum androgen, blood pressure, and triglycerides. It may also help decrease testosterone and improve IVF outcomes.

Check Your Vitamin D

Three out of four women with PCOS have a vitamin-D deficiency. This may exacerbate the symptoms of PCOS and increase the risk for multiple sclerosis, inflammation, type 1 diabetes, osteoporosis, high blood pressure, heart disease, insulin resistance, and breast and other cancers. A vitamin-D deficiency may be caused by a genetic variation or a nutritional deficit.

Vitamin D works to inhibit inflammation. In a recent study, researchers at National Jewish Health found a DNA receptor specifically for vitamin D. They discovered that a lack of vitamin D will cause suboptimal activation of the receptor and put patients at risk for inflammatory diseases. Moreover, they discovered improvement with vitamin D supplementation. Since vitamin D is critical to the absorption of calcium, a deficiency causes a cascade of related issues.

I encourage all women to have their vitamin D levels checked right away. It is a simple test, and a deficiency is usually a straightforward thing to fix and can make a world of difference throughout your body. If your doctor does recommend a supplement, choose one like PCOS Diva Super D, which combines a high-quality vitamin D with vitamins K_1 and K_2 to facilitate absorption.

Medications. Many medications sap your nutrients. Women with PCOS are almost always prescribed either the *birth control pill, metformin,* or both. Each of these depletes important nutrients, which must be replaced.

Studies show that women who use the birth control pill have lower levels of B_2, B_6, B_{12}, and folate compared to women who do not use oral contraceptives. This is of particular concern, because the body needs these critical B vitamins for metabolizing fats, proteins, and carbohydrates, and deficiency can cause anemia and depression. In fact, low levels of B_6 may explain the increased risk of blood clots in women who take the pill. Low folate can cause birth defects. Other studies indicate that the pill may deplete vitamin C, vitamin E, magnesium, selenium, zinc, and coenzyme Q. Unfortunately, zinc and magnesium deficiencies are a common cause of unexplained infertility and recurrent miscarriages. Hair loss is often an indicator of a zinc deficiency.

Meant to lower insulin levels, metformin also depletes the body of Vitamin B_{12} and other nutrients in 30 percent of patients. B_{12} has recently taken center stage, and rightly so, as a shortage of B_{12} is associated with nerve pain, cognitive dysfunction, and anemias. B_{12} is also critical for many of the detoxification pathways and for DNA stability.

Recommended Supplements

There is no "PCOS supplement." Every woman is unique. That said, there are a few supplements that I strongly advise women with PCOS to try. These supplements are certainly not the only ones that can help, but they are a good place to start. For a more complete list of supplements appropriate for women with PCOS, visit PCOSDiva.com /supplements and download the Complete Supplement Guide. Before beginning any supplements, natural or otherwise, check with your doctor for any possible interactions.

A multivitamin: A highly bioavailable multivitamin, like my PCOS Diva Essentials multivitamin, containing methylated B vitamins and insulin sensitizers such as chromium, vanadium, alpha-lipoic acid, zinc, and magnesium will support your metabolism. I take six capsules of PCOS Diva Essentials per day, three in the morning and three at lunch.

A prenatal vitamin: If you are thinking about getting pregnant, already are pregnant, or are breast-feeding, you need a high-quality prenatal vitamin. Be sure it contains folates (not folic acid), calcium and magnesium (for healthy bone development), iron, zinc (for reducing the risk of preterm birth), and iodine (for reducing the risk of birth defects).

Fish oil (an omega 3 with EPA and at least 1000 mg DHA): Most important for us, fish oil promotes normal insulin production and a healthy inflammation response. It can also support healthy hormone balance, reproductive functions, cholesterol and blood pressure levels, mood stability, and heightened brain function. Also critical is fish oil's role in our natural detoxification process by supporting the liver. If you are allergic to fish, consider an algae-based DHA supplement. I take two capsules of PCOS Diva Ultra DHA a day.

Vitamin D with K_1 and K_2: The combination of D, K_1, and K_2 is a powerhouse critical for inhibiting inflammation, boosting immunity, and supporting healthy insulin and estrogen levels and bone and artery health. Combining these vitamins enables efficient absorption. Have your levels tested before beginning vitamin D. Many women need very high initial doses in order to get a healthy and maintainable baseline. I take 4000 IUs of PCOS Diva Super D in the summer and increase it in the winter to keep my levels optimized.

Inositols: I suggest a combination of myo-inositol and D-chiro-inositol in accordance with the balance found naturally in the body. Together, these inositols manage blood-sugar levels and menstrual cycles, support your hormone and lipid levels, and promote egg quality. Each day I take two packets of Ovasitol, which is a combination inositol supplement.

A probiotic: Probiotics are well known for maintaining gut health, helping with nutrient absorption, and stimulating the immune system. They work by introducing strains of helpful bacteria to your intestinal tract. Choose a high-quality probiotic and swap brands periodically to vary the mix in your gut.

Magnesium: Women with PCOS are nineteen times more likely to be magnesium deficient than their peers. Magnesium can promote insulin regulation as well as bone and heart health. It can help ward off inflammation, depression, and anxiety as well as help muscles relax and induce sleep. For the latter reason, I suggest taking this supplement at night. I take 500 mg of chelated PCOS Diva Super Magnesium before bed.

During the Healing PCOS 21-Day Plan, I suggest the following supplement regimen:

Breakfast Supplements

- 2–3 capsules PCOS Diva Essentials Multivitamin (or similar multivitamin)
- 1–2 capsules PCOS Diva Ultra DHA (or similar fish-oil supplement)
- 1–2 droppers PCOS Diva Super D (or similar vitamin-D supplement)
- 1 sphere PCOS Diva Probiotic Sphere (or similar probiotic)
- 1 packet Ovasitol (or similar inositols supplement)

Lunch Supplements

- 2–3 capsules PCOS Diva Essentials Multivitamin (or similar multivitamin)

Dinner Supplements

- 1 packet Ovasitol (or similar inositols supplement)

Evening Supplements

- PCOS Diva Super Magnesium (or similar magnesium supplement)

How to Choose Supplements

You may have heard people argue that supplements are a waste of money. Sadly, this is often the case. Low-quality "supplements" dominate the market and are almost completely unregulated by the US Food and Drug Administration. This means that there are countless companies selling cheap supplements that will be (at best) immediately excreted. To find supplements that will benefit you, keep these guidelines in mind:

Choose supplements that are the most bioavailable. Your body is able to pull vitamins and minerals from foods more easily than from synthetic supplements in many cases. Be sure your supplements contain methylated B vitamins and chelated minerals whenever possible. You may have to take more than one capsule a day, and it may cost a little more, but remember, you get what you pay for. When your body can't use the ingredients in the over-the-counter supplements, they are excreted anyway.

Choose the right grade. There are three grades of supplements:

1. In the *nutritional grade* are your basic over-the-counter pharmacy or drugstore vitamins that we all took as kids. They promise to cover all your needs in one small pill (or chewy) per day. These supplements are rarely inspected to verify quality or contents. In addition, in order to pack everything into one pill, manufacturers use harder-to-digest, cheaper varieties of vitamins and minerals. Finally, they contain unnecessary fillers, binders, and dyes. Your body will excrete most if not all of these supplements.

2. In the *medicinal grade*, which you will find at a vitamin or nutrition store, are slightly upgraded versions of nutritional-grade supplements. They may or may not be third-party certified, but they likely contain fewer fillers and more bioavailable nutrients.

3. *Pharmaceutical-grade* supplements are third-party tested and typically contain the most bioavailable nutrients. They are

available through health professionals, like PCOS Diva, who understand the purpose, potency, and efficacy of each supplement.

Choose a supplement that is third-party certified. We have all heard the news reports of big box stores being forced to pull supplements from their shelves, because the contents of the bottles did not match the label. Third-party certification is your guarantee that the supplement has been manufactured properly, does not include any harmful contaminants, and the amounts of vitamins and minerals contained in each dose are consistent across each batch. Finally, check the label to be sure your supplement does not contain binders, dyes, fillers, excipients, and other unknown or unnecessary substances.

Sizzle in the Kitchen

If you want to eat well and feel good, you have to cook. This doesn't mean you can never dine out. It means that the majority of what you consume should be made from whole foods that you choose for their medicinal (and flavorful) properties. Knowing exactly what is on your plate and thinking about each element are critical.

As you practice and experiment with the recipes in the 21-Day Plan, you will become proficient in knowing which foods make you feel terrific and how to prepare them. If you aren't already a cook, don't worry. Just get started, and before you know it, you'll sizzle in the kitchen.

"Your recipes have converted my ultrapicky husband into someone who looks forward to trying new things. . . . You somehow made hell freeze over!"

—SOFIA A.

——————— ## PCOS Divas Love Dark Chocolate ———————

Many PCOS Divas are surprised to see how many chocolate recipes I have developed. I frequently add high-quality raw cacao powder or nibs or a few dark chocolate chips to my smoothies, snacks, and desserts. Not only is chocolate delicious and satisfying—it's good for you!

Look for chocolate as close to its natural state as possible. The higher the cacao content, the better. Shoot for at least 70 percent. Raw cacao is ideal. Avoid milk or white chocolate, as they are highly processed and have added ingredients. Here are some of the benefits:

People who regularly eat *dark* chocolate may have a lower body mass index (BMI). This may be because chocolate contains epicatechin, a flavanol found to help control food cravings and one that is more satisfying than other sweets. Also, high-quality dark chocolate is an indulgence relatively low in sugar.

Dark chocolate may increase insulin sensitivity (and make you smarter). Studies indicate that regularly eating dark chocolate increases insulin sensitivity, reducing the risk for diabetes, and improves cognitive function.

Dark chocolate reduces stress. Studies show that dark chocolate reduces levels of the stress hormone cortisol as well as catecholamine, the "fight or flight" hormone.

Dark chocolate is good for your heart. A study published in the *American Journal of Clinical Nutrition* shows that adding half an ounce of dark chocolate to the average American diet is enough to decrease blood pressure. In a nine-year Japanese study of more than forty-six thousand women, those who ate chocolate each week cut their risk for stroke.

Dark chocolate helps you relax. Chocolate contains tryptophan, a chemical that in the brain is used to produce the neurotransmitter serotonin. Serotonin is the "feel good" hormone; it helps you feel calm, confident, and happy.

Dark chocolate contains important minerals. Who knew that chocolate is a great source of iron, zinc, potassium, and selenium?!

||||||||||||||||||||||||||||||||||||||||||||||||||||||||||||||||||||||||||||||||||||||||

"Deprivation is the demise of all good dietary intent."

—AMY MEDLING

||||||||||||||||||||||||||||||||||||||||||||||||||||||||||||||||||||||||||||||||||||||||

Indulge a Little

The PCOS Diva lifestyle is not about deprivation and denial, and for good reason. If you are feeling deprived and denying yourself the joy of experiencing something, then you will inevitably cave in or rebel against the limitations. For the sake of your mind, body, and spirit, learn to mindfully indulge.

Choosing to indulge is not the same as binging. When you choose to indulge in food that you know is going to make you feel lousy, allow yourself a few bites and *savor* each one. Really revel in the taste, texture, and how it makes you feel.

Remember, even if you overindulge, *you are always one choice away from being back on track.* You don't have to throw in the towel for the day or wait until Monday to start over. Stop. Make the next choice a good one, and choose to take care of yourself.

Invest in Your Health

Have you ever heard someone say, "Your health is an investment, not an expense"? I completely agree. Your health is the soundest investment you can make. If we do not invest in ourselves with self-care, stress management, quality supplements, sleep, and healing foods, all other monetary investments we make will not really matter.

When women take on the PCOS Diva lifestyle, they sometimes get Week One sticker shock. Restocking your pantry with PCOS-friendly supplements and staples can seem daunting. A bag of apples costs more than a bag of potato chips. Initial shopping bills may be higher than you are used to. Keep in mind that you are investing money in your long- (and short-) term health. In the end, it will be way cheaper to use your produce section as a pharmacy than to make regular trips to the traditional pharmacy. Plus, you will feel good after eating the food you buy instead of feeling lousy after toting home a cartload of foods that worsen your symptoms.

To save a little money, follow sale flyers and plan menus accordingly, check out farmers' markets, club and online stores like Amazon and Thrive Market, and eat with the season.

Community Supported Agriculture

When choosing produce, try to buy local, seasonally appropriate foods. These items will typically be fresher and therefore more nutritious. I am sure you can taste the difference between a strawberry from your grocery store in February and one from your farmers' market in June. They offer completely different experiences.

Gone are the days (for most of us) of going to the butcher, the farm stand, and the local bakery. As a result, we have lost our relationship with the people and places that produce our food. We eat chemically grown tomatoes all year instead of savoring fresh ones when they are in season. We expect fresh berries in November and don't question where they came from. The result is that our bodies lose their natural seasonal rhythms, and we eat mindlessly. Fortunately, we have an alternative: Community Supported Agriculture (CSA).

A CSA is plan in which a local farmer (or small group of local farmers) offers "shares" of the weekly harvest to shareholders who pay a fee depending upon how much produce they require. Each week, the bounty of the farm is delivered to the shareholders. Some CSAs even allow shareholders to participate in the growing and harvesting of the crops.

When you take part in a CSA, you know where your food was grown, who grew it, and how. In addition, you get the absolute freshest possible produce, yielding maximum nutrition per calorie. The downside? You may not like the week's offerings, or if there are adverse weather conditions or other agricultural challenges, the harvest might be light. Personally, I think it is a small price to pay to rebuild your relationship with the origin of your food. Give it a try! For more information, check out localharvest.org.

How to Eat like a PCOS Diva

To eat like a PCOS Diva, you must first *think* like a PCOS Diva. Eating is an act of self-care and self-love. Every time you make a choice to eat something that nourishes and heals your body, you make a choice to love and respect yourself. That is how you eat like a PCOS Diva.

I often hear from women that it isn't fair that certain people can eat anything they want. Understand this: *no one gets a free pass when they eat the Standard American Diet.* The processed foods and fast food catch up with everyone. Shift your mindset to appreciate that your body sent you the warning signals to revise your eating habits, so you can undo the damage. You have an opportunity to live well in both the short and long term. Unfortunately, many others aren't listening to their bodies and will pay for it later.

We will spend the next 21 days building new skills and habits that will improve your quality of life and become your daily routine, a natural part of who you are. From how you think about food, to reading your body's signals, to dining, shopping, and planning, you will have the skills to make thriving like a PCOS Diva a sustainable lifestyle.

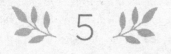

5

Move like a PCOS Diva

I have always been athletic. In my teens, I played basketball, softball, and golf. I loved moving and competing. Somewhere along the line, though, the joy I felt in movement got lost in "getting exercise." Frustrated with weight gain, I began running. Obsessively. I ran miles and miles every day, no matter what. The more I ate, the farther I ran. Any type of food indulgence was punished on the treadmill or trail. I thought I could run off the extra calories and not gain weight. I wish someone had told me it didn't work that way. Of course, exercise was burning calories, but I was damaging my body and counteracting my hard work. I never ran because I loved the way it felt; I ran because I hated the way my body looked. There was no joy in exercise, and there was little positive result. In fact, I ultimately injured myself and had to stop.

This injury was a blessing. Unable to run, I began to take walks. Guess what? The pounds slowly came off. I was no longer overtaxing my adrenal glands, muscles, and bones, and my body began to heal the damage. Moreover, with my adrenals no longer working overtime, they could get back to keeping my hormones balanced. My body felt better, my moods lifted, and I felt more like myself again.

Now I am sure to get in some movement every day. Sometimes it is a group class; sometimes it is a walk. On great days, it is playing basketball with my kids in the driveway. In my experience and that of the women I have coached, the most effective and sustainable exercise is the one you enjoy.

Movement Instead of Exercise

A PCOS Diva moves it every day. There is a big difference between exercise and movement. Exercise is something you do because you "have to." For example, "I have to go to this spin class (which I hate), or I will get fatter." Movement is something you do because it makes you feel good. For example, "I went for a bike ride today. I love the way my body feels after a good ride." See the difference?

Many of us fear that if we don't do something grueling, our bodies will not benefit. Here's a secret that will save you a lot of time, energy, and frustration. You should enjoy the movement in your day. You should feel good afterward. If you dread your daily exercise and feel exhausted and achy for days afterward, *you are doing it wrong.* Moreover, you are not doing yourself any good. Approach exercise as extreme self-care, and you'll feel the change almost right away. *PCOS Divas move every day, because we love to feel good and because we love our bodies and want to take care of them.*

Beating yourself up with exercise won't help you get healthy. Punishing yourself for how you look or what you ate is destructive—mentally and physically. For one thing, it is not sustainable. How many times have you started on an exercise routine to lose weight and then stopped after only a few weeks? That was probably because you didn't

"I don't work out because I hate my body. I work out because I love it."

—AMY MEDLING

like what you were doing. The exercise was moving your body, but not your spirit. The motivation to continue wasn't complete. If you choose movement that you love, that feeds your spirit, you will continue to do it because it feels great. Second, you are likely overtaxing your adrenal glands and making your PCOS symptoms worse.

Adrenal Fatigue

Studies indicate that 25 percent of women with PCOS have adrenal fatigue. If you are pushing extra hard, training for a marathon, or sweating it out at CrossFit and you feel as though you have been hit by a truck every morning, this may be you. The stress of your workouts might be exacerbating your PCOS symptoms and worsening your hormonal imbalances.

When you experience stress (mental or physical), your adrenal glands receive the signal to produce more cortisol (the "stress hormone") and androgens. It is the body's natural survival response to give you energy and strength to escape a predator.

Cortisol manages your body's stress response by increasing blood sugar to give you energy to run from the predator and suppressing less immediately vital functions, such as your immune system. Since women with PCOS naturally produce more cortisol to begin with, when stress is added, the problem compounds. After a period of unrelenting or chronic stress, your adrenal glands "burn out" and produce less cortisol. As a result, you feel lethargic instead of energized after a workout.

A high cortisol level creates a couple of other problems for women with PCOS. First, it raises blood sugar levels. Since most of us are working hard to balance our insulin, a cortisol imbalance can complicate the issue. Second, cortisol stores energy in fat, so that abdominal weight so many of us have only gets worse.

Stress takes an extra toll on women with PCOS, so we must find ways to manage it. One way is with movement that is pleasurable and stress relieving. If your workout leaves you feeling stressed and fatigued, it's time to switch it up. It may seem counterintuitive, but reducing the intensity of your workout will help you lose weight and feel more energized, because you calm your stress–response system. The results are lower androgens, less belly fat, and more energy!

This doesn't mean you shouldn't sweat a little! Find a way to move every day that recharges you. Try yoga or Pilates, go for a walk, do some high-intensity interval training, find a group class you enjoy, or ride your bike. If you prefer a particularly strenuous workout, go for it. As long as you feel good afterward, any movement that you enjoy is right for you. Use your self-care movement time to reduce your physical and mental stress instead of adding to it.

The Best Movement for PCOS Divas

There is no "best" movement for women with PCOS. There is only the best movement *for you*. The only requirements are that you move every day and that you enjoy the time. Otherwise, how you move is entirely up to you. Here are some suggestions for finding movement you enjoy:

Think of activities you did in your youth. Did you bike, play soccer, climb? Why not start again?

Skip the gym. There are tons of group-movement alternatives that happen outside the gym walls. Look *especially* for outdoor activity groups. Your community may have kayaking or hiking clubs, walking groups, or tai chi in the park.

Join a gym. A large commercial gym or YMCA offers a variety of activities for you to sample. The trick is to choose a facility where the staff is friendly and you feel comfortable. Take your time before making a decision. Take a tour and ask about trial memberships. If you have a friend who belongs to a gym, ask her about a guest pass.

Choose a studio. Big gym not your thing? Look for smaller studios for special activities such as kickboxing, barre, yoga, or interval training. There are also studios for women only.

As you explore the kind of movement that's best for you, consider the three types of movement that are particularly beneficial. Used in conjunction and in a way that you enjoy, they will foster weight loss, blood-sugar regulation, and mood stabilization.

High-intensity interval training (HIIT). Does "high-intensity" sound like the kind of exercise I just cautioned against as causing adrenal fatigue? It shouldn't. HIIT is a short, intense workout lasting about 15 to 30 minutes during which you alternate between levels of intensity (for example, run, jog, walk, repeat). Regular HIIT has been shown to significantly increase both aerobic and anaerobic fitness. HIIT also significantly lowers insulin resistance and results in enhanced skeletal muscle fat oxidation and improved glucose tolerance. Many gyms have HIIT classes, or you can try it on your own. It's quick, inexpensive, and the variation makes it fun. There are free apps that can guide you, including one in which you escape a zombie attack! As an added bonus, you continue to burn fat at an accelerated rate for two to twenty-four hours afterward.

Strength training. Strength training is necessary for women with PCOS for several reasons. First, muscle is metabolically active, which means it burns calories in order to sustain itself. The more muscle you have, the more calories you burn on a day-to-day basis. Second, muscle enhances your body's ability to manage glucose. Finally, feeling strong is empowering. Knowing you can open a jar by yourself or complete a hike is gratifying. Yes, as you add muscle, you will weigh more, since muscle weighs more than fat, but it takes up less space too. If you are worried about bulking up, skip the weights and use your own body weight with movements like squats and planks. Strong is the new skinny!

Mind–body movement. Many women with PCOS feel very disconnected from their bodies. We have spent so many years fighting ourselves that we are out of touch with how our body feels and what it can do. Time spent with movement like yoga, Pilates, or tai chi has the triple benefit of providing strength training, stress

Getting on Your Vagus Nerve

The vagus nerve is a major player in the parasympathetic nervous system, which is responsible for the body's "rest and digest" function. This is of particular interest to women with PCOS, because we typically have significantly higher sympathetic nerve activity, or "fight or flight" response activity.

The vagus nerve winds from your brain stem to the bottom of your abdomen, touching upon most major organs, including the heart, lungs, liver, spleen, pancreas, and digestive system, along the way. Positive stimulation of this nerve has been found to reduce inflammation. High vagal tone is associated with better blood-sugar regulation, reduced risk of stroke and cardiovascular disease, lower blood pressure, improved digestion, reduced migraines, better mood, less anxiety, and more stress resilience. Low vagal tone is associated with cardiovascular conditions and stroke, depression, diabetes, chronic fatigue syndrome, cognitive impairment, and significantly higher rates of inflammatory conditions (autoimmune disease, endometriosis, inflammatory bowel disease, etc.).

Increased parasympathetic activity via the vagus nerve improves vagal tone and improves many PCOS symptoms. Consider the following to improve your vagal tone (many of these are already part of the Healing PCOS 21-Day Plan):

- Slow, rhythmic, diaphragmatic breathing

- Humming, singing, or chanting

- Practicing yoga

- Washing your face with cold water

- Meditation

- Gargling

- Acupuncture

- Balancing your gut microbiome

relief, and an appreciation of exactly what our bodies are capable of achieving, given a little time, care, and patience. I specifically recommend yoga. Studies galore demonstrate its benefits, but a 2012 study specifically found that for young women with PCOS, it improved glucose, lipid, and insulin-resistance values. Yoga also triggers a dose of calm, probably because of its impact on the vagus nerve.

Try to engage in all three types of movement several times per week. It is easy to combine strength training with either interval training or mind–body movement. Group classes and tons of online resources are available to inspire you and help you mix it up. If you don't enjoy it, experiment and find another way.

Bonus Tip

Dress the part. Don't wait to get to your ideal shape to buy workout clothes. Well-fitting clothes that are comfortable and make you feel good make movement more enjoyable and help motivate you. You don't have to spend a fortune. My favorite yoga pants are from Old Navy!

Make a Date

Movement, just like meal planning and other self-care, must be scheduled so that it actually happens. Sit down with your calendar each week and plan when you will enjoy some self-care movement. Do not "squeeze it in." Plan around it. Make it the priority. Like breakfast, it is nonnegotiable. This mindset shift will make all the difference in how you approach movement. This is an opportunity for you to flex your PCOS Diva muscles: "No, I cannot cover for you at lunch today. I have important plans."

Once you have made the date, keep it! Treat movement like any other appointment. As the day progresses, there are always a thousand good excuses not to keep your date to move. If this sounds like you, get up early and go before the pressures of the day take hold. If you choose to move after work, don't go home! Change your clothes and get moving before the sofa calls your name. Once you get home, the mental strain of the day can make you feel more tired than your body really is. If you can get moving before that mental letdown happens, you will have more energy throughout the evening. We will work more on this in Week Two of the 21-Day Plan.

Gym Anxiety

Most every woman I work with has some sort of what I call "gym anxiety." Concerns range from not knowing how to choose a good gym, to not knowing how to use the equipment, to the most common fear, being made fun of or looked down upon. The first two are easy to fix. A quality gym will have staff willing to help get you started safely. The third is tougher and reaches beyond gym walls to most any public exercise; you might have "track," "pool," or "court" anxiety.

We all seem to have this feeling that we can't exercise where people might see us, because we aren't perfect yet and we don't belong there. No one likes the feeling of being judged and found lacking. The dread of feeling this way keeps many women from enjoying (or even making it to) the gym.

First, understand that, yes, you do belong there. The gym is for people who want to take care of their bodies and improve their lives. Everyone there is working on something (probably 99 percent of them are trying to lose weight or keep it off). A good gym will have employees and members who are encouraging and supportive. If they aren't, find a place where they are.

Second (and most important), be among the 1 percent of people who aren't breaking their necks trying to lose weight. Be the PCOS Diva who is there to practice extreme self-care. Engage in movement, whether it is at the gym, in a pool, on a trail, wherever you are, because you want to move your body so it feels good. That feeling will keep you coming back to whatever activity you have chosen and help you feel at home.

Losing weight is a byproduct of bringing yourself back into physical and emotional balance. There are lots of unhealthy skinny people. If the perfect bikini body is your ultimate goal, you will struggle to lose a pound. Feel sorry for all those miserable-looking people as you move and enjoy it. *You deserve to feel good!*

One of the best ways to beat gym anxiety? Take a buddy. It can be a lot more fun to move with a friend. You can motivate each other, share in your successes, commiserate in setbacks, and laugh when things just go wrong. Studies show that people who engage in movement with a partner have more success and move more regularly.

Sleep Is an Important Exercise

Sleep is critical to a PCOS Diva's movement plan. Obviously, you will not be able to move in an enjoyable way if you are dragging due to a lack of sleep, but there's more to it. If you are chronically sleep deprived, you are at greater risk for injury; hormones are imbalanced; your body is less able to repair organs, muscles, bones, and tissues; you make bad food choices; and you become increasingly forgetful. Several recent studies show the clear relationship between sleep, food consumption, weight regulation, and metabolism.

Did you know that people who habitually sleep less than six hours per night are more likely to have a higher-than-average body mass index (BMI)? Researchers believe that this is because our bodies secrete hormones while we sleep that control appetite, metabolism, and glucose processing. Lack of sleep can wreak serious havoc on your insulin levels, put you at higher risk for diabetes, anxiety, and depression, and worsen your PCOS symptoms, especially if you sleep less than five hours per night.

Leptin and Ghrelin

Chronically sleep-deprived people have low levels of leptin, a hormone that signals your brain when you have eaten enough food. They also have high levels of ghrelin, which stimulates appetite. Put these two together, and you have a body craving food it doesn't need, taking in sugar to boost lagging energy, and being too tired to exercise.

Millions of us are chronically sleep deprived for many reasons.

Lifestyle choices: Sleep is often the first thing to be sacrificed when we are overcommitted. Work, family, and social obligations compete for time in our day with self-care, including movement and sleep.

Disease and/or medical conditions: Many diseases and conditions make it difficult to sleep, either because you cannot get comfortable and relax or because they literally wake you, as in the case of sleep apnea. Often these diseases are caused, in part, by sleep deprivation. Diseases such as coronary disease are worsened by sleep deprivation, creating an unhealthy cycle.

Sleep apnea: Women with PCOS are at least thirty times more likely to struggle with sleep apnea than those without. It is closely linked to insulin resistance and creates a vicious cycle in which insulin resistance causes sleep apnea and vice versa. If you snore loudly and wake with a dry mouth, headaches, or shortness of breath, and if your partner observes that you stop breathing during sleep, you should be tested for sleep apnea right away. Sleep apnea will worsen your insulin resistance and glucose processing, making your PCOS symptoms worse and possibly leading to other serious health problems.

Medication: Sleep disruption is a common side effect of many popular medications. Read the label, and ask your pharmacist and doctor about the side effects of all medications, whether over-the-counter or prescription.

Melatonin imbalance: Melatonin is a powerful hormone that regulates your circadian rhythm, the cycle of waking and sleep. Disruption in its levels often results in sleep deprivation or unhealthy sleep patterns.

Cortisol imbalance: Your cortisol levels should naturally rise and fall. Ideally, they peak around 8 a.m. and drop off between midnight and 4 a.m. If you wake between 1 and 3 a.m., it may be because of low adrenal function and cortisol or inadequate glycogen reserves in the liver.

Strive to sleep seven to eight hours per night. Six hours seems to be the minimum amount of sleep the average person needs per night to function and be healthy. More than eight and a half to nine hours can also create metabolic issues. Here are some tips for getting a good night's sleep:

Eat the right foods. During the day, choose foods that promote sleep (potassium-rich fruit, dark leafy greens, turkey, whole grains), and avoid sleep-interfering foods (anything high in fat or sugar—even natural sugars like berries). If blood sugar drops below 50 mg/dL at night, it can increase levels of adrenaline, glucagon, cortisol, and growth hormone, all of which can stimulate the brain. But eating a big meal before sleep is not a good idea either. Your body will be too busy digesting to focus on the restorative aspects of sleep, like detoxifying, regenerating cells, and reviving. If you must eat before bed, the best snacks contain both a carbohydrate and the amino acid tryptophan. Legumes, nuts, and seeds are all good choices. Apples and nut butter or a little gluten-free, oat-based granola with nuts and coconut milk are my go-to choices for a before-bed snack.

Support your adrenal glands. Although cortisol helps your body to adjust to perceived emergencies, chronic stress can lead to adrenal fatigue, a cortisol imbalance, and sleeplessness. Consider supporting your adrenals with a high dose of rhodiola, licorice root, ashwagandha, ginseng, and maca root. My PCOS Diva DeStress supplement is a terrific herbal combination, and it can help. Also, take steps to manage your stress during the day. Experiment with relaxation techniques, yoga, and daily movement.

Supplement with magnesium. Magnesium is the "relaxation mineral." Unfortunately, women with PCOS are nineteen times more likely to be deficient than the average person. Leafy green veggies, oatmeal, pumpkin seeds, black beans, and almonds are all good sources of magnesium. You can also choose a high-quality supplement or take an Epsom-salt bath. Adequate magnesium doesn't guarantee a good night's sleep, but lack of magnesium will literally keep you up at night.

Boost your melatonin. Melatonin must have darkness to trigger activation (even if it is supplemented). Turn off lights and pull light-blocking shades (I swear by my sleep mask). Turn off electronics at least an hour before bedtime.

Practice a sleep ritual. A sleep ritual is a crucial element for ensuring a good night's sleep. Relax your body and mind for 30 to 60 minutes before bedtime to signal your body that it is time to sleep. It gives your mind time to settle so it isn't racing and making "to-do lists" and helps your muscles to let go of the stress of the day. Try to go to bed at the same time each night. Turn off electronics at least an hour before bed, and practice letting the stresses of the day melt away. Repeat the same steps every night before bed, and your body will begin to anticipate going to sleep. This will be part of your 21-Day Plan.

Cut back (or cut out) caffeine, stimulants, and sugar, especially after lunch. Don't consume caffeine four to six hours before bed. This includes dark chocolate!

Avoid alcohol. Don't drink alcohol for several hours before sleep. If you have a glass of wine to help you sleep, it will initially act as a sedative, but it disrupts REM (rapid eye movement) sleep, and you'll wake up in the middle of the night when the alcohol is being metabolized. Stick with a drink at dinner if you must, three hours or so before bedtime.

Try sleep-inducing herbs. Valerian root is one of the most studied herbs connected with sleep. It increases receptors for gamma-aminobutyric acid (GABA), a neurotransmitter that is involved in regulating normal sleep. Chaste tree, or *Vitex*, may increase body's production of melatonin during the night too. Lemon-balm tea can calm a restless mind and is effective for easing anxiety.

Breathe. Focused breathing helps reduce your heart rate and blood pressure, releases endorphins, and relaxes your body, getting you ready for sleep. Try the Box Breath: Inhale for 4 counts, hold for 4 counts, exhale for 4 counts, rest for 4 counts, and repeat 4 times. We will experiment more with more breathing techniques during the 21-Day Plan.

Seek treatment if you have an underlying medical condition. A health-care professional can help you resolve sleep apnea, depression, or anxiety.

Move like a PCOS Diva

During the next 21 days, you will find a way to joyfully move every day. You will experiment with types of movement and find the right ones for you. You will seek out joy in movement and find activities that make you feel good. You will discover ways to stay motivated and on track and make movement a sustainable part of your everyday life from now on. You will sleep well. While nourishing your body with the food it craves, you will treat your body as it deserves to be treated—with love, care, and respect. Movement is as critical to thriving with PCOS as changing how you think and eat. Done the PCOS Diva way, it balances your body, mind, and spirit.

PART TWO

The Healing PCOS 21-Day Plan

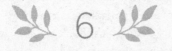

6

Prepare for Success

It's time to get started. Preparation is critical to living the PCOS Diva lifestyle. Although you cannot anticipate every contingency every day, you can lay out a plan that smooths the path to feeling great. Let's start from the inside out.

Step 1: Think like a PCOS Diva. If you skipped Chapter 3, please go back and read it now. It is the foundation of your next 21 days.

Step 2: Consider your Big Why. Why exactly are you doing the Healing PCOS 21-Day Plan? If your answer is "I want to lose weight," I urge you to look deeper. Why do you want to lose weight? So you can get pregnant or have more energy? So you can look amazing at your school reunion and make people eat their cruel words? Whatever your reason, you must be honest with yourself about it. Understanding the true Big Why of your commitment will give you a clearer goal and more satisfaction when you achieve it. If you can find the reason that emotionally resonates with you, and if you keep reminding yourself of that reason, you are more likely to overcome challenges and stick with your healing journey.

Remember my couch story? My desire to be a more engaged and active mother and wife was my Big Why. It still is. Whenever I come to an obstacle, I look at my family and refocus on my goal. Thinking of my family renews my determination and helps me over whatever road-block is in my way (and the roadblocks are always changing). When I have fallen off the wagon and just don't want to get back on, I call on my Big Why to carry me through.

Step 3: Assess the situation. When you're feeling good, it is easy to forget exactly how bad you felt earlier. This will likely be your situation in the coming weeks. The changes you are about to make will alleviate symptoms, and feeling energized and healthy will become your new normal. That's great! In order to really appreciate your future progress, take a moment and do the PCOS Diva Symptom Assessment found at the end of the book (p. 303). At the end of the 21-Day Plan, you will take it again and compare your totals. You may be surprised at how far you've come!

Step 4: Ask for help. For many of us, asking for help is difficult. We don't want to burden other people or admit weakness. Now is the time to start living like a PCOS Diva and asking for help and support. Not only do studies indicate that people who make lifestyle changes with a partner have more success; you *deserve* help and support.

Ask someone to engage in the 21-Day Plan with you. Together, you can prepare, support, and thrive! Alternatively, you can gather a group, or "PCOS posse," to support you. Try explaining to a few key people at home and at work what PCOS is, why you are taking on this new lifestyle, and exactly how they can support you. Be specific and clear. "Please take a walk with me at lunch" or "Please don't bring bagels to my desk." And remember to express gratitude for their assistance and enthusiasm for the process.

As your energy levels rise and your moods lift, people will begin to notice the change. Soon, instead of asking for help, you will be inspiring others.

Step 5: Clean out your pantry. It's time for a clean slate. Today, you will begin to eliminate all the foods that are making you sicker. Donate or throw away processed foods. This includes pastas, cookies, and snacks. If they aren't in your kitchen, it will be harder for you to fall back into old eating habits. As a rule of thumb, get rid of anything with ingredients that you do not recognize or cannot pronounce and anything with more than five ingredients on the label. Especially get rid of anything containing:

High-fructose corn syrup. An inexpensive sweetener with a high glycemic index, high-fructose corn syrup not only alters your metabolic rate to encourage fat storage, but increases the risk for type 2 diabetes, coronary heart disease, strokes, and cancer.

Trans fat or partially hydrogenated oil. Hydrogenated fats are highly processed and used to make foods last longer and have a less greasy feel. You'll find them in margarine, vegetable shortening, commercially baked goods, deep-fried foods, and fast foods. If a label has "partially hydrogenated" listed in any of the ingredients, toss the product. The FDA allows companies to label a product with .49 percent or less of trans fat per serving as 0 percent grams of trans fat.

Artificial sweeteners. Artificial sweeteners go by many names, including aspartame, acesulfame potassium, Equal, NutraSweet, and sucralose. Although these sweeteners do reduce calories, they slow your metabolism, and some have been shown to increase your cancer risk. They have also been linked to metabolic syndrome disorders like PCOS and general toxicity.

Refined sugar. Virtually all processed food contains refined sugar in some form. Consumption of high amounts of (often hidden) sugar and the corresponding elevated insulin levels can cause weight gain, bloating, fatigue, arthritis, migraines, lowered immune function, obesity, cavities, and cardiovascular disease. It can also disrupt absorption of nutrients, possibly leading to osteoporosis, depression, and PMS symptoms.

Monosodium glutamate (MSG). MSG is a flavor enhancer that can stimulate appetite and cause weight gain. Many people experience a host of other side effects such as headaches, itchy skin, dizziness, and respiratory, digestive, circulatory, and coronary concerns. You will often find MSG in restaurant food, salad dressing, chips, frozen entrees, and soups. In addition to MSG, there are other ingredients that contain the offending chemical found in monosodium glutamate (processed free glutamic acid) that causes adverse reactions; these should be avoided as well: autolyzed yeast, maltodextrin, calcium caseinate, yeast food, glutamate, hydrolyzed protein, monopotassium glutamate, sodium caseinate, textured protein, yeast extract, and yeast nutrient.

Benzoate preservatives (TBHQ, BHA, and BHT). Benzoate preservatives are often added to foods to preserve fats and keep them from becoming rancid when they age and are exposed to light and air. They prolong shelf life and are also used as a defoaming agent. They are a weak estrogenic and have been shown to affect sleep and appetite. Benzoates are associated with metabolism and nutrition disorders, liver and kidney damage, and cancer.

Brominated vegetable oil (BVO). BVO is most often used to keep flavor oils in suspension in citrus-based soft drinks. It has been banned in one hundred countries (though not the US) because it can interfere with reproduction, alter thyroid hormones, and impair neurological development.

Sodium nitrate and sodium nitrite. Preservatives often used in processed meats, such as bacon, jerky, sausage, hot dogs, and luncheon meats, nitrates can increase your risk of heart disease. They may also affect the way your body uses sugar, making you more likely to develop diabetes, and can combine with chemicals in the stomach to form nitrosamine, a highly carcinogenic substance.

Artificial flavors and colors. Artificial flavors and colors are linked to allergic reactions, dermatitis, eczema, asthma, some cancers, hyperactivity and ADHD in children, and nerve damage. In addition, they can contain up to 10 parts per million of lead and 3 parts per million of arsenic and still be generally recognized as safe by the FDA!

Genetically modified organisms (GMOs). GMOs are plants and animals that have been genetically modified to be larger, have better color, or be disease or pest resistant. Since virtually all American corn, soybean, cotton, and canola crops have been modified, ingredients made from them are found in most processed food. There is concern that these GMO products, once consumed by humans, may cause antibiotic resistance or have a negative impact on our genetic functions. Engineered plants may be less prone to disease and pests and thus need less insecticide and pesticide, but if modified genes escape into the wild, pest and/or disease strains with greater resistance may develop that will require larger doses of these toxins to keep them in check. Until we are certain of the long-term implications of GMOs, try to avoid them whenever possible.

When buying canned goods, look for BPA-free cans. BPA (bisphenol A) is an endocrine disruptor often found in can linings (and many other places) that can worsen your symptoms.

Step 6: Restock your pantry. We will restock your pantry with PCOS Diva essentials. This list is long. I do not expect you to buy everything on the list immediately. This is your ultimate pantry. Take a look at the Week One Meal Plan at a Glance (p. 133) to see what you will need right away. Your pantry will slowly fill with healing foods.

Beverages (unsweetened): seltzer, herbal teas, green tea, coconut water, filtered water, sparkling mineral water

Condiments: coconut aminos, olive-oil mayonnaise, stone-ground and Dijon mustards, tamari soy sauce, Worcestershire sauce

Dried herbs, spices, and flavorings: allspice, bay leaf, black pepper, cardamom, cayenne pepper, celery salt, chili powder, Chinese chili paste, cloves, cinnamon, coriander, cumin, curry, pure extracts (almond, coconut, lemon, peppermint, and vanilla) garlic powder, ginger, nutmeg, onion powder, oregano, paprika, smoked paprika, whole peppercorns, rosemary, thyme, Himalayan salt, sea salt

Flours: finely ground almond flour, arrowroot, coconut flour, gluten-free all-purpose flour (use sparingly), gluten-free baking mix (use sparingly)

Grains: amaranth, buckwheat, millet, gluten-free rolled oats, gluten-free steel-cut oats, quinoa, brown rice, wild rice, gluten-free bread crumbs

Nuts (raw nuts are less inflammatory than roasted): almonds, Brazil nuts, cashews, hazelnuts, macadamia nuts, pecans, pine nuts, pistachios, walnuts, nut butters

Oils and vinegars: organic grass-fed butter, ghee, avocado oil, virgin coconut oil, flaxseed oil, hemp-seed oil, medium-chain triglyceride (MCT) oil, extra-virgin olive oil, sesame oil, walnut oil, raw apple cider vinegar, white and red balsamic vinegar, red-wine vinegar, rice vinegar

Seeds: chia seeds, flaxseed, hemp seeds, pepitas (shelled pumpkin seeds), poppy seeds, sesame seeds, sunflower seeds, seed butters, tahini

Smoothie supplement powders, essentials: fiber (such as PCOS Diva Power Fiber), protein (such as PCOS Diva Power Protein or Power Vegan Protein) (see box on p. 106)

Smoothie supplement powders, extras: greens (such as PCOS Diva Power Greens), reds (such as PCOS Diva Power Reds), L-glutamine, matcha tea powder (see box on p. 106)

Snacks (for more snack ideas, see pp. 294–98): dark chocolate, unsweetened shredded coconut, Mary's Gone Crackers, unsweetened dried fruit, coconut manna

Sweeteners:

Stevia. Stevia is a natural sweetener that is two to three hundred times sweeter than cane sugar; a little goes a long way. Watch out for inexpensive varieties that use alternative sweeteners as filler. Look for organic green stevia powder.

Raw honey. Raw honey has a glycemic index of only 40 to 55, is totally natural, and is recognized for its antimicrobial properties.

Depending upon the source, it can range in flavor and color. Be sure to buy only pure honey.

Maple syrup. Also completely natural with a glycemic index of 54, quality maple syrup contains only pure tree sap. Avoid brands containing added ingredients like corn syrup.

Monk fruit. The intense sweetness (two to three hundred times sweeter than refined sugar) of monk fruit, also known as Buddha fruit, comes from antioxidants. The sweetener naturally has zero calories and doesn't increase blood sugar.

Coconut sugar. The major component of coconut sugar, with a low glycemic index and rather unique taste, is sucrose (table sugar). Although coconut sugar has a marginally lower amount of the monosaccharide, make sure you don't consume more than you would of table sugar.

Avoid agave nectar (syrup). It has a high concentration of fructose and, once processed, loses all nutritional value.

Vegetarian proteins: black beans, kidney beans, chickpeas, lentils, lima beans, mung beans, pinto beans, white beans, yellow beans, nut butter (almond, cashew, hazelnut), seed butter (sunflower, pumpkin seed, tahini)

Other: canned coconut milk, canned pumpkin, cacao powder, canned chopped green chilies, sundried tomatoes in olive oil, organic chicken and beef bone broth, organic vegetable stock, canned diced tomatoes, tomato paste, tomato sauce

Step 7: Ready your kitchen. Cooking is easier and more enjoyable when you have an efficient space. First, eliminate kitchen clutter, including gadgets and appliances that you don't really use. I suggest doing this in small increments. Spend 15 minutes a day; choose one cabinet, drawer, or countertop and declutter it.

——— Choosing Smoothie Supplement Powders ———

Essentials

Fiber. Look for powders that contain fiber from a variety of sources with a balance of soluble and insoluble fiber and are gluten and lectin free and high in antioxidants.

Protein. When choosing a protein powder, be sure to select one that is gluten, dairy, soy, and GMO free. PCOS Diva protein powders are formulated with the nutritional needs of women with PCOS in mind and are either collagen- or organic pea protein–based. If you choose to shop around, I highly recommend choosing a soy-free, vegan, or collagen powder that is unsweetened or slightly sweetened with stevia.

Extras

Greens. Your greens powder should not contain gluten, bulking agents or fillers (such as fiber, whole grasses, pectin, rice bran, or flax), added sugars or artificial sweeteners, or alfalfa (contains a toxic element shown to aggravate autoimmune disease).

Reds. Choose a reds powder that is free of soy, sugar, and artificial sweeteners. It should not contain gluten or bulking agents or fillers (such as fiber, whole grasses, pectin, rice bran, or flax). The reds powder should combine well over a dozen fruits and vegetables and their phytonutrients from the red/purple group.

L-glutamine. Choose a pure L-glutamine powder with no fillers that is made from non-GMO ingredients.

Matcha tea powder. Matcha is a powerful antioxidant. Since you are ingesting the entire tea leaf, make sure your matcha tea powder is ceremonial grade, organic, free from pesticides and heavy metals, and non-GMO.

Next, reorganize. Be sure to place all commonly used tools and ingredients near each other. Then move lesser used items to peripheral storage areas. Set aside dedicated space and materials for meal planning.

Finally, restock. You will be cooking up a storm, and the right tools can make this easier and more enjoyable. Here are small appliances and gadgets I suggest:

- Quality cookware. Cast iron and stainless steel are best. Try to avoid Teflon nonstick whenever possible. If you aren't ready to give up nonstick, go with ceramic.
- A powerful blender that can crush ice and pulverize greens. I use a Vitamix. It's expensive, but I've found it works the best. I also like the NutriBullet Pro and use this when I travel.
- An immersion blender. Great for making soup.
- Good-quality chef's and paring knives.
- A spiralizer. Not essential but recommended.
- A slow cooker.
- An electric pressure cooker.
- A mini slow cooker. Great to bring to work to heat leftovers, soups, oatmeal.
- A rice cooker. In addition to cooking rice, it is great for cooking oatmeal in the morning.

Step 8: Gather your self-care tools. You will need the following:

- A 1-inch three-ring binder
- A natural-bristle dry brush or loofa with a detachable long handle so you can brush your back
- A tongue scraper
- A water bottle (glass or stainless steel)
- An attractive journal and your favorite pen
- Sleep mask
- Sticky notes
- Supplements (to select and order, see p. 73)

Filter Your Tap Water

Filtering your drinking water is very important, since women with PCOS are more susceptible to endocrine disrupting chemicals (EDCs) that are commonly present in drinking water. These EDCs can disrupt your hormones and worsen your PCOS symptoms.

Carbon filtration is the most common type of water filter and is highly effective at removing water contaminants such as chlorine, pesticides, herbicides, polychlorinated biphenyls (PCBs), volatile organic compounds (VOCs), some pharmaceuticals, and disinfection byproducts. Simple systems like Pur or Brita are easily found and affordable.

Other water-filtration systems include reverse osmosis, ion exchange, steam distillation, ceramic filters, ultraviolet, and Berkey. Each system has its strengths and weaknesses. If you would like to invest in a high-end water-filtration system, check out my favorite, AquaTru's counter-top water purifier.

Do your research and choose the system that is right for you. Start with a water analysis. In the US, you can get a copy of your local Community Confidence Report or your local Water Quality Report at www.ewg.org/tap-water/.

Step 9: Make a plan. *Meal and snack planning is critical to success.*

Weeks One and Two of the Healing PCOS 21-Day Plan have suggested meal plans and recipes. During Week Three, you'll prepare your own meal plan based on what you've learned. Before each week begins, allocate some time to plan for the next four days or so of meals and snacks. Look over the week's meal plan and decide if you need to make any substitutions or rearrange meals for your preference or convenience. Make a list of the necessary groceries and shop. On the third or fourth day, plan and shop for the rest of the week. This twice weekly shopping will become a habit for you once you get in the swing of living like a PCOS Diva.

Meal and snack prep is an important part of your self-care. Having the right ingredients on hand and foods prepared ahead of time can eliminate the temptation to order takeout or fall back into bad food habits. I have learned a few tricks over the years to making meal planning easy. Now I can plan a week ahead in 20 to 30 minutes. Here's how:

Recognize that meal planning is an important part of self-care. Prioritize time to sit down, look through recipes, and make lists. Have a cup of tea, relax, and make this an enjoyable time that is scheduled for supporting your health. Time spent planning, shopping, and cooking is an investment in you!

Make a date with your calendar. Sit down on the weekend and figure out how much time you have each night to make dinner. Do you have time for a sit-down meal, or will it be a quick dinner on your way back out the door? If you know time will be short, consider a slow-cooker meal or something you can prepare (at least mostly) the night before. Bear in mind that things don't always go as planned. Sometimes you work late, get stuck in traffic, or have a long day and just don't want to deal with dinner. Don't worry, get frustrated, or beat yourself up. I will teach you how to plan for these occasions too.

Check to see what you already have. Take a look in your refrigerator and pantry. What's left? Do you have anything that needs to be used up?

Check sale flyers. If grass-fed beef is on sale, add it to the week's menu. Wild-caught salmon looks good? Buy double and freeze half. When basics or expensive items go on sale, stock up and store or freeze what you can.

Rate Your Menus

After each meal, rate it on a scale of 1 to 5. Meals earning 4s and 5s go back into rotation; 1s through 3s get tossed. Make notes on each recipe to help you remember the adjustments you'd like to make next time, for example, "Use less lemon."

Make a shopping list. Make a detailed list of everything you need for the week, from breakfasts through dinners (including snacks and replacement of staples). Consider keeping a template list of basics you buy every week that you can simply add items to and go. This may eliminate return trips, saving you time and money and preventing impulse buying. *Never* go to the store without a list.

Shop smart. Start at the farmers' market. The produce will be fresher, more nutritious, and probably cheaper. Then move on to the grocery store. Learn when the perishables get stocked. Fish comes in every day except Monday? Great; plan around that. Also, be flexible with your list. If the spinach looks a little wilted, but the asparagus looks great, switch it up.

Plan for "planned-overs." Leftovers aren't left over if they are planned. Plan to have a little extra left after a meal so you can enjoy it for lunch the next day. Alternatively, plan to use it in a recipe later in the week. For example, I love to make roast chicken.

Bonus Meal Prep Tips

Hard-boiled eggs will last one week in the refrigerator. They are a quick, flexible, portable protein.

Make a batch of steel-cut oatmeal for the week. This is a fantastic breakfast for PCOS Divas. Make a batch, store it in an airtight glass container in the refrigerator, and just scoop out a serving in the morning. It reheats in a flash with a dash of nondairy milk.

Smoothies store like a dream. Smoothies are my go-to breakfast. Make a large batch and freeze it in muffin tins. When you're ready, pop a few into the blender. Alternatively, measure out all the dry ingredients and freeze or refrigerate them in storage bags. When you're ready, add your nondairy milk and blend!

Your slow cooker is your friend. Every slow cooker is different, so you will have to play around with cooking times. I like to keep ingredients on hand in my pantry and freezer for a few slow-cooker meals. Depending upon the recipe, I prep the recipe in the morning and put the ingredients in my slow cooker, and it is ready at dinnertime. Serve with a green salad for a complete meal.

An electric pressure cooker makes fast food. I love my pressure cooker. It took a short time to master, but now it is one of my most-used shortcuts. I can make gorgeous and nutritious dinners in a fraction of the conventional cooking time.

It is great the first night, but sometimes it's even better later in the week on a salad or in soup.

Have a backup plan. A well-stocked freezer and pantry can save you when things go awry. Redefine fast food for these occasions. For example, frittatas are quick, easy, and can usually be made with whatever is on hand. Freeze marinated meats for quick meals, or grill and freeze protein ahead of time for salads. I will often make double batches of entrées or side dishes and freeze one. This works especially well for soups, stews, rice, and quinoa. On a hectic night, thawing soup or stew is faster than ordering takeout!

Prep on the weekend. Spend a little time on the weekend washing and chopping up veggies, frying ground meats, making soups, and washing up fruits and vegetables. You can even set up your salads in jars a few days in advance.

Step 10: Prepare time and space. Each morning, you will start your day with time set aside just for you. During Week One, you will journal during this time. During Weeks Two and Three, you'll add movement and meditation. Spend a few minutes now and prepare a space where you can journal and work through your morning routine. Put your journal, pens, and sticky notes in the space.

Step 11: Start detoxing from processed foods and caffeine. If your current diet includes caffeine and processed foods, you may experience a detox period in which you have headaches, a feeling of malaise, and cravings as you transition to PCOS Diva–friendly foods and beverages. Before you begin the Healing PCOS 21-Day Plan, begin reducing your intake of these foods, especially caffeinated drinks, sugar (including artificial), and processed food.

Step 12: Trust the process. During the first week you will experience highs and lows as your body finds balance, you adjust to new habits, and your mind learns to calm itself. Trust that everything is happening

The Healing PCOS 21-Day Plan is not a short-term diet. It's a powerful way to live!

the way it should. Live in the moment, and make one choice at a time. I promise that at the end of the 21 days, you will feel like a new woman. Most important, your body will be stronger and healthier.

So right now, let go of doubts that may linger. Release doubts that this will help you achieve your goals. Release doubts that you have the inner strength to stick with it. Let it all go and give yourself over to the power of the process. You will not regret it.

Tips for Surviving Caffeine Detox

- Cut your dose of caffeine in half every day until you are down to ½ cup and then stop.
- Drinking water and healthy snacking throughout the day can help to crowd out coffee and caffeine.
- For help with headaches, take 1000 mg of vitamin C during this time to help lessen the withdrawal symptoms.
- White willow bark tablets, which contain a natural type of pain-relieving salicylate, can also help with headaches. Like aspirin, however, willow should be avoided for two weeks before and after surgery.
- Even if you quit cold turkey, most symptoms should disappear after one week.
- If you must have a little caffeine, have a cup of green tea.
- Drink warm water with lemon or switch to lower-caffeine green, white, matcha, or oolong tea.

What to Expect During Week One: Discover

In Week One, we will lay the groundwork for the habits, patterns, and motivations that are the foundation of the PCOS Diva lifestyle, which will be yours for the rest of your life. There is a secret to learning to live as a PCOS Diva: *baby steps*. The incremental steps you take throughout your day, every day this week, will change your health and your life.

"The PCOS Diva lifestyle has changed my health in dramatic ways. I went from being tired and depressed (despite trying multiple antidepressants) to more energetic and motivated. I was thrilled to see positive results so quickly, like weight loss and a decrease in my acne. I suddenly had a wealth of information and support at my fingertips that made me feel so empowered and motivated to tackle my PCOS. I didn't make a lot of changes all at once—I started with what I could handle and slowly added more changes when I was ready and as I started to feel better. Treating PCOS isn't a one-and-done thing—it's a lifestyle that you maintain and build upon throughout your life. You can do it!"

—KATIE B.

The Healing PCOS 21-Day Plan will help guide you through these small steps as they become new positive habits.

This first week is focused upon how you will become a PCOS Diva. The habits you begin building this week will become so integrated into your routine that they become a fundamental part of who you are. As you feel better and better, these healthy habits will become self-perpetuating.

Your goals for the week are to:

- Discover how you can take charge of your health by taking charge of your day.
- Discover how food makes you feel.
- Discover how to think like a PCOS Diva.

Above all, this week and always, be kind to yourself. *We are striving for progress, not perfection.*

Here are the elements of your new daily healing and renewal routine.

Rocket Launch

Taking control of your day begins with rising *on purpose with purpose.* The rising is the important part. How many times do you wake up, only to hit the snooze button? Do you lie in bed and ruminate over all the things you have to do today? Anxiety, procrastination, and negative thoughts simmer until you drag yourself out of bed at the last possible moment. You start your day already in a rush, skip breakfast, and head out the door frazzled and frustrated with yourself.

That is not the way a PCOS Diva takes on her day. You are about to discover a better way.

Adopting a regular and consistent wake time is a powerful way for you to take charge of your life and your health. Just the act of waking up and rising earlier feels like a victory. It becomes an act of self-care because you create space and time in your day just for you. Please make the commitment right now not to hit the snooze button.

It all begins with getting out of bed 15 minutes earlier than you normally do. Ideally, by the end of the program, I would like you to rise about 45 minutes earlier. This will be critical self-care time that will allow you to start your day on the right foot. So if you want to increase that amount of time a little each day to get you to your end goal gradually, then please do!

Each morning, you will "rocket-launch" yourself out of bed using speaker and author Mel Robbins's "5 Second Rule." Essentially, as soon as the alarm rings and before your brain has time to realize what is happening, you say to yourself, "5–4–3–2–1—LAUNCH" and get yourself out of bed.

In her book *The 5 Second Rule*, Robbins says, "If you have an impulse to act on a goal, you must physically move within 5 seconds or your brain will kill the idea." If you are like me, when that alarm goes off, you can typically come up with five good arguments for why you deserve to hit that snooze button, but if you just rocket-launch yourself out of bed without thinking, then there is no time to argue or negotiate.

So rise and shine, PCOS Diva!

Morning Motto

For most of us, the first thing we do in the morning is grab our phones and start scrolling through email, texts, and social media. This is an anxiety-inducing way to begin your day. Please don't look at your phone until at least breakfast. Instead, as soon as your feet hit the floor, proclaim your intention for the day, your Morning Motto.

Your Morning Motto should be something that is easy to remember, a phrase that can become your guidepost and motivation for the day. It can anchor you when you feel as though you are drifting, inspire you to take action, and help you overcome obstacles, persevere, and keep moving forward.

Lately, I have been using the morning motto of Pam Grout, the author of *Thank and Grow Rich*: "Something amazingly awesome is going to happen to me today," coupled with Philippians 4:13 ("I can do all things through him who strengthens me"). I also love, "Take in the good," a wonderful motto from Rick Hanson's book *Just One Thing*. These mottos help me start my day focused on possibilities and abundance.

Find your own Morning Motto for the next 21 days and write it down in your journal before you begin Day 1. You can make one up, use something from your favorite devotional or inspirational book, or even search the internet for ideas. Here are some to get you started:

- "Good habits make a PCOS Diva."
- "Surrender to yes."
- "Just breathe."
- "I think I can."
- "Health first."
- "There is no failure, only feedback."
- "Progress, not perfection."

Big Why

Take a moment to remember your greater motivation, your "Big Why," for becoming a PCOS Diva. Reminding yourself of your ultimate goal can make the day's choices (like getting out of bed earlier) a little easier.

Gratitude

Begin your morning with a grateful heart and it will set a positive tone for the day. Make a short mental list of things you are grateful for at this moment. They don't have to be profound. Some days, I am grateful for the peaceful silence of the morning before the house wakes and the hustle of the day begins. Be grateful for the power to make decisions that change your life. Be grateful for your cozy slippers. It doesn't matter if it is large or small, just start the day with gratitude.

Morning Elixir

After you rocket-launch out of bed, proclaim your Morning Motto, and spend a few moments with your Big Why and gratitude, it will be time to have your morning elixir. Starting your day, at least 30 minutes before breakfast, by drinking a cup of warm water with lemon is a wonderful way to hydrate first thing in the morning. Lemon water helps to "wake up" your GI tract and prepare it for the act of digestion; as a result, the body is better able to absorb nutrients and bloating is reduced. It is also a great way to show your liver some love. Lemons, more than any other food, boost the liver's capacity to produce enzymes. Both water and lemon juice help the liver to function more efficiently and improve your overall health. Finally, lemons are a good source of antioxidants and electrolytes like potassium, calcium, and magnesium.

To make your morning elixir:

- Bring your tea kettle to a boil.
- Squeeze the juice of a quarter to a half of a lemon in a mug.
- Fill your mug halfway with filtered cold water.
- Fill the mug the rest of the way with hot water.

Consider adding one or more of the following:

Cayenne (dash). A sprinkle of cayenne will wake you up with a little kick, and the capsaicin in cayenne may help to regulate your blood-sugar levels. Studies have shown that it increases the temperature of your body and kick-starts your metabolism, reduces appetite, and helps break down fats.

Fresh ginger (1 teaspoon). Ginger has anti-inflammatory compounds called gingerols and can also support blood sugar. I like to grate a little ginger root, put it in a tea ball, and let it steep in my lemon water.

Raw apple cider vinegar (1 teaspoon). A teaspoon or two of apple cider vinegar can help improve insulin sensitivity. (Remember, if you are on metformin, consult your doctor before ingesting apple cider vinegar.)

Ground cinnamon (¼ teaspoon). Numerous studies have shown that cinnamon can lower blood glucose and even glycated hemoglobin (HbA1c). I use Ceylon cinnamon rather than the cassia type. Cassia cinnamon contains coumarin, which could be harmful to the liver. Ceylon cinnamon has no measurable amount of coumarin.

Ground turmeric (¼ teaspoon). Turmeric is a bright yellow-orange spice that is part of the ginger family. Curcumin, the active ingredient in turmeric, may alleviate inflammation.

Raw honey (½ teaspoon). If you must have a little sweetener, use a locally sourced raw honey. Studies have shown that it can help with diabetes, sleep problems, coughs, and wound healing.

Inspiration

Contemplating meaningful and inspirational quotes has changed the way I approach life. It is a tool that has helped me to think like a PCOS Diva. These quotes act as little nuggets of wisdom that bring light and hope and often touch my soul. They can awaken a sense of faith, perseverance, and strength. They sometimes help me to see life from a whole new perspective. Reading and reflecting upon a meaningful daily quote is a powerful way to change our thinking; it can help us see something in ourselves that we want to change or overcome.

So while the water is boiling for your morning elixir, take a moment to reflect on the Inspiration quote. What does it mean for you in your life? How could you apply it to your day?

Affirmation

Positive affirmations have helped me to think like a PCOS Diva. They have helped me to replace the limiting ideas, negative beliefs, and sabotaging self-talk that had become part of me and my story. Positive affirmations have helped me to become aware of my thoughts and shift the internal dialogue that often tells me I'm not enough toward positivity, gratitude, and "enoughness." Throughout our lives we have received so many negative assertions, either implicitly or explicitly; we were told by a parent, coworker, classmate, or teacher that we didn't have the ability, that we were fat, lazy, stupid, and so on. These negative assertions are not "truth," but they have the power to stay with us. Positive affirmations can work to crowd them out, so we don't continue to reinforce them.

During the next 21 days, I will give you a positive Affirmation for each day. If it doesn't resonate with you, please feel free to write your own.

Each morning, you will write the daily affirmation three times on three separate sticky notes and put the sticky notes in three locations where you will see it throughout your day. I like to place one on my bathroom mirror (saying your affirmations out loud while looking at yourself in the mirror is extremely powerful), one in the middle of my car steering wheel, and one on my computer monitor.

Think about the best locations for your sticky notes. Maybe in your wallet, makeup bag, or desk drawer would be more discreet. The trick is to find a spot that will trigger you to say the affirmation to yourself. Every time you see the affirmation, say it to yourself three times. If you don't feel comfortable leaving the affirmations out in the open, set an alarm on your phone to ring three times each day, and then say your affirmation to yourself. Try to get into the feeling of the affirmation. If the affirmation is "I am healthy and radiant," work on *feeling* healthy and radiant while you say it.

Dry Brushing and Oil Massage

Every morning for the next 21 days, take 3 minutes to use your new natural-bristle brush to do some "dry brushing" before you take your morning shower. Use your brush to apply firm but gentle pressure on your skin. It should feel good!

Dry brushing is a wonderful act of self-care. It is a way to energize and wake us up in the morning while we are caring for and getting in touch with our bodies. It stimulates our lymphatic system, rejuvenates and invigorates us, and supports detoxification, one of the major functions of our skin. Brushing the skin also helps unclog the pores, increase its ability to absorb nutrients, and increases circulation to the skin cells. The nervous system is rejuvenated, and nerve endings are stimulated. After dry brushing and a shower, I recommend applying a body oil (I like organic untoasted sesame oil for its warming qualities). You'll feel soothed and centered for the day ahead.

Those with eczema, acne, or other skin problems should consult with a health practitioner before dry brushing.

How to Dry-Brush
Always brush in the direction of the heart.

1. Start with your right foot. Brush in a circular motion first on the outside upward, then the inside, working your way up to the top of the leg. Repeat on the left leg.
2. Skip the stomach because brushing there can cause nausea.
3. Brush the right buttock, then the left in a large circular motion, ending with strokes upward.
4. Brush the right hand and arm as described for the legs: outer first, then the inner area, working upward. Repeat on the left arm.
5. Brush the ribs from the top down to the waist.
6. Brush the back from the neck area downward, moving horizontally (or with circular motion if this is difficult).

Then take your normal shower. If you can tolerate it (I can't), alternate between warm and cool water, ending with cool water, to really boost circulation.

Lightly pat the skin with a towel, leaving it rather moist. Finish by taking a couple of minutes to massage in nourishing oils that are absorbed quickly into the skin such as untoasted sesame, coconut, or almond. After you have stimulated the skin's nerve endings with the brush and the shower, the oil provides a calming sensation.

Breakfast and Supplements

If you can't wait for breakfast, have it before you dry-brush and shower. Just be sure to eat breakfast. Remember, you are breaking your fast from the night before and keeping your blood sugar even. Take your morning supplements with breakfast.

Tongue Scrape

After breakfast, brush your teeth and use a tongue scraper. I know it may sound a bit gross, but trust me, it will help curb cravings and may help with digestion, stimulate internal organs, and reduce bad breath. It is just another good habit to help crowd out the negative habits. Notice how it helps, particularly with evening cravings, when you scrape after dinner.

Diva Daily

Each day throughout the Healing PCOS 21-Day Plan, I will give you a Diva Daily lesson that draws upon the Think, Eat, or Move principles of being a PCOS Diva. Please make sure you set aside 15 minutes in your day to read the Diva Daily lesson and take action on the Diva Do.

Diva Do

Diva Do activities are designed to help you to Think, Eat, or Move like a PCOS Diva. They will reinforce and complement the Diva Daily lesson. You may not be able to complete the entire activity in the

15 minutes allotted. That is okay. Know that you can always come back to it. Remember, "Progress, not perfection."

Morning Snack/Tea Time

You may find that you don't need to have a snack in the morning, especially since your new breakfast habits should hold you until lunch. Experiment and discover your personal regimen. Skip this snack if you are having an early lunch. At least take a moment to make yourself a cup of tea, a glass of water, or another PCOS Diva beverage.

Lunch, Supplements, and Walk

We will focus on creating a movement mindset throughout this program. In Week One, you will start by taking a 15-minute walk after

---

Savor Your Chocolate

A little bit of dark chocolate a day makes the cravings for sweets go away. During the 21-Day Plan, give yourself full permission to enjoy a bit of high-quality dark chocolate (a square or two) every day. This isn't a snack—it's a mindful indulgence. The chocolate should be at least 70 percent cacao. Cacao is the number one food source of magnesium and chromium, which really help with cravings.

Don't just gobble it down without tasting it. Be very mindful when you eat your chocolate. Try to experience it with all of your senses.

Look at your chocolate and notice the color. *Smell* the rich aroma. *Hear* the sound the chocolate makes when you snap it in two. *Feel* the texture on your fingers.

After looking, smelling, and snapping, nibble off a small piece of the chocolate with your front teeth and take it into your mouth. Resist the urge to chew and eat. Instead, hold the chocolate against the roof of your mouth and pass your tongue over the bottom of it, noticing first how it melts and then how it feels. Now finally *taste* your chocolate.

This is how we mindfully enjoy something decadent and delicious. We do it intentionally, taking in the pleasures with all of our senses. This is mindful indulgence.

---

lunch (and/or dinner). This will increase your energy to take on the afternoon, and a brief walk after a meal may improve digestion and blood-sugar control. You will also take your lunch supplements.

Afternoon Snack/Tea Time

An afternoon snack is nonnegotiable. One of the toughest times to stay productive during the day is between 2 and 3 p.m. There is no denying the mid-afternoon sluggish feeling that occurs almost every day for most people. We need to be especially careful to keep our blood sugar balanced and energy up with a snack and hydrate with water or tea. Be sure to do a water check. Have you had enough water today? If not, hydrate now. You don't want to catch up too close to bedtime.

Dinner, Supplements, Walk, and Prep for Tomorrow's Meals

Each evening, you'll make dinner, eat, take a walk, and prep for the next day's meals and snacks. You will also take your dinner supplements.

Nighttime Ritual

I used to plop myself in front of the TV at night with a bag of chips or bowl of ice cream and stay up late watching shows I didn't really enjoy. I'd often be too tired to drag myself to bed and just fall asleep on the couch, way too late, only to be exhausted the next day. The lack of good-quality sleep was wreaking havoc on my PCOS.

In order to take charge of my PCOS, I had to take charge of getting myself out of bed in the morning *and* of putting myself to bed at a reasonable hour, relaxed and ready for sleep. I had to change my habits and establish a new nighttime ritual.

During the next 21 days, you will work out your own Nighttime Ritual, creating a predictable routine that allows you to unwind, helps to settle your thoughts, and gets you ready to drift off to sleep. Create your own ritual using the following components.

UNPLUGGING

Create more space in your life for peace and positivity by unplugging from media—all social media, phones, TV, and computers—by 8 p.m. Doing so also reduces your exposure to artificial light before bedtime. Charles Czeisler, a top sleep expert and director of the Division of Sleep Medicine at Harvard Medical School, finds that spending time in front of screens before bed increases the metabolism and reduces the release of melatonin, a hormone responsible for regulating sleep. A recent study showed that those who read on a tablet before bed had reduced levels of melatonin, took longer to fall asleep, and spent less time in restorative REM sleep. In addition, tablet readers reported being sleepier and less alert the following morning, even after eight hours of sleep, and they experienced a delayed circadian rhythm.

Ideally, remove devices from your bedroom entirely. If you now use your phone for an alarm clock, please purchase and use a traditional alarm clock instead. If you absolutely have to do work on a computer or check your phone before bed, install an app that reduces blue light in the evening.

EVENING ELIXIR

I find that preparing and sipping on a cup of something warm and soothing keeps me out of the pantry and away from evening munching. I especially like Spiced Almond Milk. Here are some of my favorite evening elixirs for you to try. These teas all contain relaxing, sleep-inducing herbs:

- Nighty Night Tea from Traditional Medicinals
- Sleep and Relax Tea from Gaia Herbs
- Soothing Caramel Bedtime Tea from Yogi Tea
- Nighttime Tea from Pukka
- Snore and Peace Tea by Clipper

Spiced Almond Milk

Makes 1 serving

1 cup unsweetened almond milk
1 teaspoon raw honey
¼ teaspoon ground cinnamon
Dash of ground cardamom
Dash of ground nutmeg
Dash of ground ginger
¼ teaspoon pure vanilla extract
1 tablespoon almond butter

Heat all ingredients in a small saucepan until steaming. Pour into blender and blend for 30 seconds, leaving the hole on top open for steam to escape. It will be nice and frothy, like a coffeehouse latte.

SMALL BEDTIME SNACK

See if having a small bedtime snack works best for you. You don't want to wake up in the middle of the night due to low blood sugar. Most nights, if I go to bed before 10 p.m., I try to fast from dinner to breakfast the next day. However, if I feel my blood sugar dip before bed, I will have a small snack, typically a few apple slices and nut butter or ⅓ cup low-sugar nut granola (Bear Naked Fruit and Nut is my favorite) with coconut milk.

TOMORROW'S PRIORITY LIST (TPL)

I used to spend most of my time before I drifted off to sleep thinking about all I had to do in the morning. Then when I woke up, I would lie in bed thinking of all I had to do that day. It would cause a lot of anxiety and make me feel overwhelmed. My secret to drifting off to a restful sleep is having this all out of my head.

During your bedtime ritual, allot time to jot down all of your to-dos for the next day. Do you need to go to the post office? Buy a present for grandma's birthday? Make a dentist appointment? Whatever it is, get it down on the list and out of your head. Then create a second list of five things you will accomplish tomorrow. This short list is your TPL. Put it on an index card, and you can start your day tomorrow knowing your priorities. Be sure to remember to add self-care to the list. Don't forget to cross off the items on your list as you accomplish them. There is simple satisfaction gained in checking off a job done.

MAGNESIUM

Magnesium helps relax muscles, which may be one reason it helps prepare us for sleep. Magnesium also helps to activate GABA receptors, which exist across all areas of the brain and nervous system. GABA is a calming neurotransmitter that the brain requires in order to switch off; without it we remain tense and our thoughts race, when we should be shutting down for sleep. Without adequate magnesium, we are unable to effectively activate GABA receptors and utilize GABA effectively. Magnesium can also help reduce cortisol, which can keep you up at night.

Here are some ways to get a little extra nighttime magnesium:

Oral magnesium supplement. Bedtime is a great time to take your magnesium supplement. I mix a teaspoon (300 mg) of PCOS Diva Super Magnesium in water.

Epsom-salt or magnesium-salt detox bath. During the course of the next 21 days, take at least one detox bath. Epsom-salt baths can provide magnesium sulfate transdermally. Alternatively, you could use "magnesium salt" or magnesium chloride.

Detox Bath

Makes enough for 1 bath

2 cups Epsom salt
½ cup baking soda
10 drops lavender essential oil
5 drops geranium essential oil
3 drops clary sage essential oil

Magnesium oil. Magnesium oil is made by combining magnesium chloride flakes with water. Spray a little on your hand and rub it over your arms and legs.

ESSENTIAL OILS

Essential oils will help you to relax before bedtime. I love to add them to a detox bath or footbath. You can also use a diffuser to scent your bedroom during your bedtime routine. Use carrier oil to dilute essential oils before applying them to your skin, since undiluted essential oils applied directly may cause skin irritation. I like to rub a little on the back of my neck and shoulders or on the bottoms of my feet.

Lavender is one of the most studied oils and has been shown to help with mild insomnia.

Bergamot, known for its ability to relieve anxiety and tension, is found in Earl Grey tea (one of my favorites for its soothing properties).

Ylang-ylang activates the alpha-wave activity in the back of your brain, which leads to relaxation and helps you sleep more soundly.

Clary sage is one of my all-time favorite oils for PCOS. It can help decrease cortisol levels and acts like a natural antidepressant.

Valerian, **vetiver**, and **Roman chamomile** also have a calming effect.

STRETCHING

Stretching before bed is one of the best ways to unwind after a long day. It helps to release muscle tension and allows you to focus on your body and your breath. Stretching can be an active meditation, allowing the mind to calm. Commit to five different stretching poses before bed. Check out YouTube or Pinterest for ideas.

READING A BOOK

You read a bedtime story to a child. Why not read one to yourself? Researchers at the University of Surrey (UK) found that stress levels were reduced as much as 68 percent just by reading, especially before bed. Sometimes moving into a fictional world is a great escape and prepares our consciousness for a dream state. The trick is to find a book that you can put down and isn't a page-turner that will keep you up until 3 a.m. And don't use a device that emits blue light!

GRATITUDE STONE

A gratitude stone is a small rock that you can carry in your pocket as a reminder to be grateful. I found a smooth, oval rock on Footbridge Beach in Ogunquit, Maine. It is one of my favorite places, and I always feel joy and gratitude when I am there. This stone sits on my bedside table, and every night before I go to sleep, I pick up the smooth stone in my hand and think of one thing that I am thankful for from my day. Ideally, begin and end your day with gratitude for the abundance of blessings you currently have in your life. Bringing more gratitude into your life will have a tremendous positive impact on your healing journey and help you discover your PCOS Diva.

SLEEP MASK AND LIGHTS OUT BY 10 P.M.

Get into bed and be ready for sleep by 10 p.m. Cortisol levels are supposed to drop at nighttime, allowing your body to relax and recharge. If your cortisol levels are too high, you may find that even if you've been exhausted all day, you get a second wind or cortisol surge at night, especially when you are up past 10. We want to reduce cortisol at night, not elevate it! Retrain your body.

My bedroom window faces the street, and if I want to have my window open for a cool breeze, the street light shines right in my eyes. Since I've started using a sleep mask, I've found I sleep deeper, and I now can't sleep without one. Eye masks and sleeping masks function by covering the light receptors within the eyes, signaling the body to produce the sleep-inducing hormone melatonin. Trust me, get a sleep mask and use it!

Final Thoughts as You Begin Week One

Plan to begin on a Monday. That will give you the weekend before to shop and prepare. Preparation is the key to success, so start off right!

You may experience fatigue and low levels of energy, headaches, malaise, and/or runny nose. This is most likely during the first few days while your body gently detoxes and adjusts to a new way of eating. As the week goes on, and especially around Day 4, you will have increasing energy.

You may experience an emotional release at unexpected times. Some of the Diva Do exercises may trigger unexpected emotions. Think of emotions as energy in motion. In order for the emotions to pass through you and move on, you must feel them fully and not shut them down. You can accomplish this by writing in a journal, drawing, talking to a friend, or any method that works for you. The important thing is to process the emotions that come up and then let that energy move on. Often simply feeling and acknowledging your feelings is enough to let them go.

On some days you may feel heavier than usual, and on others you may feel lighter, but by the end of the week you should feel less bloated and may even lose some weight. This program isn't just about the weight, though, and I invite you to put the scale away for the week (or longer). Don't let a machine dictate the way you feel about yourself.

You may have some mood swings and food cravings as your body adjusts to this new way of eating. You may also feel a bit off, perhaps uneasy or lethargic. Don't worry; this is just your body detoxing. Keep drinking lots of water. Trust me, by the end of the week you will feel great.

Approach the week ahead with an open mind. If you encounter a food that you have never tried before, give it a shot. If you don't like it at first, try and try again. It has been shown that you may need to try a food nine or ten times before you like it. If you are not going to use my recipes due to time, cost, or preference, please create a meal plan of your own using the approach outlined in Chapter 4, "Eat like a PCOS Diva," to create simple meals with lots of seasonal produce.

Keep in mind that we are working toward progress, not perfection. When you can't resist that bagel in the break room or have that extra glass of wine, don't beat yourself up. Relish the indulgence. Then make the next choice one that will help you feel good in both the short and long term.

Savor and reward your successes. When you make a good choice, spend a moment to congratulate yourself and acknowledge your progress.

The most important preparation you can make for Week One is to work on your mindset. When you begin to think like a PCOS Diva, you will naturally act like a PCOS Diva. Remember, *you deserve to feel good.* The Healing PCOS 21-Day Plan is just the beginning of your journey toward thriving.

One Last Prep Tip

Don't binge the day (or week) before you start the program! It is totally unnecessary. There are no foods that are absolutely off-limits. It isn't as though you will never taste ice cream again.

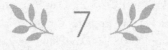

7

Week One:

DISCOVER

Welcome to Week One!

You have taken the first big step and committed to upgrading your lifestyle and healing your PCOS. The week ahead will be full of ups and downs and new discoveries about yourself. One day, you will look back on this week and feel proud of yourself and grateful that you began this leg of your journey. You will surely wish you had started sooner. So let's get going!

First things first. Remember our mantra, "Progress, not perfection." It is so important, as you enter into the next 21 days and beyond, to focus on this simple phrase. The Healing PCOS 21-Day Plan provides an ideal. Adjust it as necessary to work for you. Do your absolute best and be satisfied with that. Inevitably, you will have the occasional slipup. That's okay! We are striving for slow, sustainable change.

When things don't go as planned, remember, you are only one choice away from getting back on track. It is okay if your alarm clock doesn't go off and you miss your morning routine. Just keep moving forward, take a deep breath, and make your next choice a positive one. Don't wait until tomorrow to begin again. Soon you will discover your rhythm and what works (and doesn't work) for you!

Week One Weekend Prep: Get a Running Start

You will start the Healing PCOS 21-Day Plan on a Monday in order to have the entire weekend to prepare. On Saturday and Sunday before you begin the Healing PCOS 21-Day Plan:

- ☐ Look over the Week One Meal Plan at a Glance (p. 133). Do you need to make any substitutions or rearrange the meals to fit your schedule? Using the Meal Plan and the meal-planning tips in Step 9 of Chapter 6 (p. 108), plan your food for the week.
- ☐ Based upon your Meal Plan, make a detailed list of the grocery items you need for the week, from breakfasts through dinners, including snacks and replacement of staples. Look in your pantry and refrigerator. What do you have on hand and what do you need to put on your shopping list for the next four days?
- ☐ Grocery shop for the next three or four days.
- ☐ Prepare and package snacks for Week One that can be made in advance, for example, Sweet Spiced Pepitas (p. 294) and Pumpkin Spice Protein Bars (p. 241).
- ☐ Wash, chop, and store veggies for snacks and salads for the first three or four days.
- ☐ Make homemade Hummus (p. 292; if not using store-bought).
- ☐ Make a batch or two of White Balsamic Vinaigrette (p. 286).
- ☐ Be sure you have all of your self-care items (see Chapter 6, Step 8, p. 107).
- ☐ Review the Week One Daily Protocol (p. 136), so you know what to expect.
- ☐ If you haven't already, complete the PCOS Diva Symptom Assessment (p. 303).

🌿 Week One Meal Plan at a Glance

Monday, Day 1

Breakfast	Snack (Optional)	Lunch	Snack (Required)	Dinner
Apple Pie Smoothie (p. 229)	⅓ cup shell-on pistachios	Layered Lunch Wrap (p. 252) with Hummus (p. 292)	½ sliced avocado sprinkled with sea salt and lime juice with 6 Mary's Gone Crackers	Garlic Roasted Chicken (p. 270), Roasted Roots (p. 277), Orange Roasted Brussels Sprouts (p. 277), and mixed greens with White Balsamic Vinaigrette (p. 286)

Tuesday, Day 2

Breakfast	Snack (Optional)	Lunch	Snack (Required)	Dinner
Avocado, Egg, and Arugula Rice-Cake Breakfast Toast (p. 239)	1 small sliced apple with 2 tablespoons sunflower-seed butter, sprinkled with hemp or chia seeds	10-Layer Salad in a Jar (p. 248) with chicken and White Balsamic Vinaigrette (p. 286)	⅓ cup Hummus (p. 292) and vegetable crudités	Rich and Creamy Chicken Stew (p. 255) and mixed green salad with White Balsamic Vinaigrette (p. 286)

Wednesday, Day 3

Breakfast	Snack (Optional)	Lunch	Snack (Required)	Dinner
Apple Cobbler Super-Seed Quick Oats (p. 236)	1 hard-boiled egg and vegetable crudités	Planned-over Rich and Creamy Chicken Stew and mixed greens with White Balsamic Vinaigrette (p. 286)	¼ cup Sweet Spiced Pepitas (p. 294)	Veggie Tacos (p. 267) with Gingered Apple and Apricot Slaw (p. 282)

Thursday, Day 4

Breakfast	Snack (Optional)	Lunch	Snack (Required)	Dinner
Chocolate Cherry-Berry Smoothie (p. 230)	¼ cup Sweet Spiced Pepitas (p. 294)	10-Layer Salad in a Jar (p. 248) with organic deli-style smoked turkey and White Balsamic Vinaigrette (p. 286)	1 Pumpkin Spice Protein Bar (p. 241)	Lentil Soup (p. 260) and Dani's Mediterranean Chopped Salad (p. 282)

Friday, Day 5

Breakfast	Snack (Optional)	Lunch	Snack (Required)	Dinner
1 Pumpkin Spice Protein Bar (p. 241)	⅓ cup shell-on pistachios	Planned-over Lentil Soup and mixed greens with White Balsamic Vinaigrette (p. 286)	⅓ cup Hummus (p. 292) and vegetable crudités	Maple-Mustard Salmon (p. 272), Whipped Butternut Squash (p. 278), and Garlicky Greens (p. 278)

Saturday, Day 6

Breakfast	Snack (Optional)	Lunch	Snack (Required)	Dinner
Overnight Blueberry Buckle Steel-Cut Oats (p. 238)	1 small sliced pear with 2 tablespoons sunflower-seed butter, sprinkled with hemp or chia seeds	10-Layer Salad in a Jar (p. 248) with salmon and White Balsamic Vinaigrette (p. 286)	1 hard-boiled egg and vegetable crudités	EAT OUT

Sunday, Day 7

Breakfast	Snack (Optional)	Lunch	Snack (Required)	Dinner
Lemon Poppy-Seed Pancakes (p. 245)	¼ cup Sweet Spiced Pepitas (p. 294)	10-Layer Salad in a Jar (p. 248) with organic deli-style smoked turkey and White Balsamic Vinaigrette (p. 286)	celery sticks and 2 tablespoons cashew butter with 5 dried cranberries	Grass-fed sirloin steak with Chimichurri Sauce (p. 288), Grilled Cauliflower Steaks with Sweet Vidalia Onions (p. 281), and foil-packet sweet potatoes (4-Step Grilled Veggies, p. 280)

Discover: Week One Daily Protocol

Rocket Launch. *Wake up 15 minutes earlier than usual.*
- ☐ Morning Motto
- ☐ Big Why
- ☐ Gratitude

Morning Reflection
- ☐ Morning elixir
- ☐ Inspiration
- ☐ Affirmation

Shower
- ☐ Dry brushing before shower
- ☐ Oil massage after shower

Breakfast
- ☐ Meal
- ☐ Breakfast supplements
- ☐ Tongue scrape

Daily Lesson
- ☐ Diva Daily
- ☐ Diva Do

Morning Snack/Tea Time
- ☐ Optional snack
- ☐ Beverage break

Lunch
- ☐ Meal
- ☐ Lunch supplements
- ☐ 15-minute walk

Afternoon Snack/Tea Time
- ☐ Required snack
- ☐ Beverage break
- ☐ Water check (have you had enough water today?)

Dinner
- ☐ Meal
- ☐ Dinner supplements

- ☐ 15-minute walk
- ☐ Dessert chocolate (optional)
- ☐ Next day food prep

Nighttime Ritual
- ☐ Unplugged by 8 p.m.
- ☐ Evening elixir and/or evening snack (only if needed)
- ☐ Tomorrow's Priority List
- ☐ Magnesium
- ☐ Tongue scrape
- ☐ Essential oils
- ☐ Stretching
- ☐ Book
- ☐ Gratitude stone
- ☐ Sleep mask and lights out by 10 p.m.

Food Prep for Monday, Day 1

- ☐ Prepare and package snacks.
- ☐ Prepare Garlic Roasted Chicken (you can season the chicken in advance and leave it in refrigerator until ready to roast).
- ☐ Peel and chop root veggies for roasting.
- ☐ Trim brussels sprouts for roasting.
- ☐ Prepare Layered Lunch Wrap with Hummus (put it together in the morning to take to work; if it sits overnight, it will get soggy).

🌿 Day 1

Meal Plan

Breakfast	Snack (Optional)	Lunch	Snack (Required)	Dinner
Apple Pie Smoothie (p. 229)	⅓ cup shell-on pistachios	Layered Lunch Wrap (p. 252) with Hummus (p. 292)	½ sliced avocado sprinkled with sea salt and lime juice with 6 Mary's Gone Crackers	Garlic Roasted Chicken (p. 270), Roasted Roots (p. 277), Orange Roasted Brussels Sprouts (p. 277), and mixed greens with White Balsamic Vinaigrette (p. 286)

Inspiration

"Do not wait until the conditions are perfect to begin. Beginning makes the conditions perfect." —Alan Cohen

Affirmation

"My courage is stronger than my fear."

Diva Daily

"What we eat, we become." Take a moment to reflect on this phrase, and you'll realize its truth. It reflects the relationship between food and health: when you put good in, you get good out. The nutrients in our food determine the makeup of our cells and our hormones. If the average woman has to replace around 300 billion cells every day, then the foods we eat are the building blocks of the cells that will replenish us.

It isn't enough to know that we are what we eat; we have to take it a step farther and feel the effect of the foods we choose. We have to get in touch with, in a very mindful way, how food makes us feel, both physically and emotionally. This one thing can literally change our life and put us in a place of power and control.

Instead of following the latest diet fad or conventional nutrition wisdom, *follow your body's wisdom.* Listen to what your body is telling you. It really is as simple as that.

Diva Do

Use your journal throughout the 21-Day Plan to jot down how you feel before and after you eat every meal and snack. Think of this Diva Do assignment as collecting data for a science experiment. You are experimenting with how food makes your body feel, so of course you need to collect data. But just like a good scientist, you are going to be objective and collect the data with curiosity and without judgment. If you go completely off program and eat a donut for breakfast, don't beat yourself up with shame, guilt, and regret. Merely make an observation about how you feel after you've eaten it and record it in your journal.

You will use the data you collect to make more powerful decisions regarding the food you put in your body. We are looking for the food that makes us feel vital, alive, energized, balanced, centered, and just plain good.

In your journal, write down the time and what you ate. Take note of how you felt physically and emotionally before, right after eating, and again two hours later. Sit quietly after you eat and reflect. Note how your energy level, your moods, and your physical symptoms are affected by the food in your body. Bodily sensations are physical responses to foods.

Physical Signs of Imbalance or Inflammation

- Headaches
- Stomach pain
- Nausea
- Bloating
- Constipation
- Diarrhea
- Muscle cramps

- Coughing
- Runny nose
- Fatigue
- Insomnia
- Restlessness
- Shakiness
- Muscle weakness
- Poor concentration
- Brain fog
- Pallor

Physical Signs of Balance

- Bright eyes
- Hunger for next meal or snack
- Stamina
- Natural deep breathing
- Good digestion
- High energy
- Restful sleep
- Focus
- Alertness
- Strength
- Good attention span
- Good color

Emotional responses may be a little harder to notice.

Emotional Signs of Imbalance

- Anxiety
- Negativity
- Feelings of emptiness or lack
- Boredom
- Fear
- Anger
- Sadness
- Depression

- Absentmindedness
- Restlessness
- Irritability
- Agitation
- Hyperactivity
- Edginess

Emotional Signs of Balance

- Cheerfulness
- Positivity
- Feelings of wholeness and abundance
- Confidence
- Excitement
- Energy
- Playfulness
- Happiness
- Enthusiasm
- Focus
- Calm
- Flexibility
- Patience

At first it may feel a little weird to get in touch with your bodily state, either physically or emotionally, after eating; or you may not feel any particular way. That's okay; just write "fine" or "good." But the more information you can gather, the better you will be able to get in touch with how food is making your body feel. Do whatever you can to make this process quick, easy, and sustainable for the next 21 days. If it is easier to keep this information on a notepad on your mobile device, please do!

Remember, this experiment is designed to be informative. *Stay free of negative judgments.* If negative feelings arise, or if you feel guilty for eating something "bad," remember that recording this information will help you to see the connection between what you eat and how you feel physically and emotionally. At the end of the week, you will analyze the data.

Food Prep for Tuesday, Day 2

- ☐ Prepare and package snacks.
- ☐ Cook three hard-boiled eggs (one for tomorrow's breakfast and the others for snacks later in the week).
- ☐ Set remaining chicken aside for Rich and Creamy Chicken Stew and 10-Layer Salad in a Jar with chicken.
- ☐ Prepare 10-Layer Salad in a Jar with chicken.
- ☐ Prepare Homemade Chicken Bone Broth for Rich and Creamy Chicken Stew. I like to make it in a slow cooker on low overnight and then strain and store it in the refrigerator in the morning.

Day 2

Meal Plan

Breakfast	Snack (Optional)	Lunch	Snack (Required)	Dinner
Avocado, Egg, and Arugula Rice-Cake Breakfast Toast (p. 239)	1 small sliced apple with 2 tablespoons sunflower-seed butter, sprinkled with hemp or chia seeds	10-Layer Salad in a Jar (p. 248) with chicken and White Balsamic Vinaigrette (p. 286)	⅓ cup Hummus (p. 292) and vegetable crudités	Rich and Creamy Chicken Stew (p. 255) and mixed green salad with White Balsamic Vinaigrette (p. 286)

Inspiration

"Life's not about expecting, hoping, and wishing; it's about doing, being, and becoming. It's about the choices you've just made, and the ones you're about to make. It's about the things you choose to say—today." —Mike Dooley, www.tut.com

Affirmation

"I free myself from destructive habits."

Diva Daily

It is time to take charge of your lab tests and results. For so long, I would take myself out of the process at the doctor's office, especially when it came to blood tests. I would take the order to my lab without any understanding of what was being done. I would wait for the nurse to call and tell me, "Everything looks good" or "Your testosterone is high," and that was the extent of my involvement in the process. If that sounds like you, then that stops today. PCOS Divas know that knowledge is power. The more we understand about our bodies and our unique brand of PCOS, the better we can translate the signals our body sends and contribute to our own healing. So today you will begin to take control, track, and understand your health care.

Diva Do

Today you will begin building a Lab Binder. If you don't already have your labs for the last three years, pick up the phone, call your doctor, and request that the office send you hard copies of the last three years of your lab work. You will keep hard copies of all of your labs in the three-ring binder you selected during prep, along with any other doctor's notes you receive.

Then spend a little time today becoming familiar with the labs I recommend in the PCOS Diva Recommended PCOS Labs Guide. Download it at PCOSDiva.com/labs. Get to know the names, purpose, and ranges of relevant tests. These are tests that you should advocate for when you visit your doctor.

For instance, many women with PCOS have undiagnosed hypothyroidism and often Hashimoto's disease. Many doctors will only test thyroid-stimulating hormone (TSH) levels, which doesn't give you the whole picture of what is going on with your thyroid. You will have to ask for more tests.

Also, the majority of women with PCOS are vitamin-D deficient, and again, doctors won't always test vitamin-D levels. Optimizing these levels can make a huge difference in the way you feel. Remember it is important to be a PCOS Diva at the doctor's office!

Once you receive the hard copies of your tests, put them in your binder, and from here on out, always ask for hard copies to store in your binder. It is affirming to see the progress you make. For example, I can look back at my labs over time and see how my total testosterone (the range for this is 6–86 ng/dL) went from a 70 to 16! Seeing your lab results improve is validating to you and your doctor, who really speaks the language of labs.

Food Prep for Wednesday, Day 3

☐ Prepare and package snacks.

☐ Package planned-over Rich and Creamy Chicken Stew and mixed-greens salad for lunch.

☐ Shred 4 cups cabbage and 1 carrot for tomorrow's Gingered Apple and Apricot Slaw and store in refrigerator.

☐ Chop 1 zucchini, 1 yellow summer squash, 1 green bell pepper, 1 red bell pepper, and 1 onion into ½-inch pieces for tomorrow's Veggie Tacos and store in refrigerator.

🌿 Day 3

Meal Plan

Breakfast	Snack (Optional)	Lunch	Snack (Required)	Dinner
Apple Cobbler Super-Seed Quick Oats (p. 236)	1 hard-boiled egg and vegetable crudités	Planned-over Rich and Creamy Chicken Stew and mixed greens with White Balsamic Vinaigrette (p. 286)	¼ cup Sweet Spiced Pepitas (p. 294)	Veggie Tacos (p. 267) with Gingered Apple and Apricot Slaw (p. 282)

Inspiration

"Old patterns will flare up when you commit to new ways of being."
—Danielle LaPorte

Affirmation

"I can do this."

Diva Daily

You may not even recognize destructive old patterns until new habits start to crowd them out, but today you are going to really become aware and mindful of old patterns creeping back in.

One of the old patterns I had to contend with was eating in secret. I would deny myself anything pleasurable in public; I would eat something I considered a "forbidden food" in secret and then feel shame and guilt afterward. For instance, I would often, at the very last second at the grocery store, throw a Snickers bar on the conveyor belt. The cashier would ask if I wanted to keep it for my purse. I would grumble assent, not making eye contact, and grab the bar. I would eat the bar in a few bites in the car on the way home, hide the wrapper, and try to pretend the whole thing never happened. I ate in secret most often when I was feeling angry, sad, or stressed, and the food was a way to numb my negative emotions for a very short time. The sugar would give me a buzz, acting as an instant pick-me-up. But it was always short-lived and always followed by a blood-sugar crash and lots of shame, guilt, and regret.

I think my eating in secret stemmed from living a deprivation and denial lifestyle. Since I was constantly on some form of restrictive diet, my ego would rebel. It would say to me, "What do you mean I can't have a Snickers?" However, once I allowed myself anything I wanted, my ego would calm down, and I wouldn't want the Snickers so much. The secret was in the allowing.

As you move through the 21-Day Plan, you will become more aware of these old negative habits, whether they are dietary, mindset, or behavioral.

Diva Do

If this story resonates with you and you are a secret eater, make the commitment to stop now. The remedy is in allowing. Allow yourself to feel pleasure. PCOS Divas don't eat in secret. We know that food has the power to nourish and is meant to be pleasurable, and you are definitely not enjoying it if you are hiding in the bathroom to eat it. Let go of the shame over how you eat, what you eat, and how you feel because of it. Food is nothing to be ashamed of, and guess what? Neither are you!

Is there another old pattern flaring up? How can you quell it or crowd it out with a new habit? Be aware of your triggers. Do you eat junk when you are bored or procrastinating? Did you hit the snooze button today because you didn't prep for Day 3? Today, do two things.

Notice your old patterns and triggers, and write them down in your journal. My trigger was a grocery cart full of "diet" food that didn't really feed my body and soul. Diet frozen dinners and sugar-free, fat-free yogurt were not satisfying. Perhaps I reached for the Snickers bar because I was unconsciously responding to the marketing tagline "Snickers satisfies."

Create a new habit for each old pattern or trigger, and write what you will do in your journal. Now when I go to the grocery store, I make sure to purchase something that is on the Healing PCOS plan, and is also satisfying. Now I get a delicious bar of NibMor cherry chocolate every week. I no longer feel compelled to eat it in secret or stuff it down on the way home. Rather, I save it for when I can mindfully enjoy it.

The trick is to be mindful of your pattern triggers. You may need to call upon the 5–4–3–2–1 rocket-launch strategy to go with the new habit for a while (before your mind talks you out of it). It will take some conscious effort here to reprogram those old patterns into healthier new ones. The important thing is to forgive yourself if you slip up, and make adjustments. Remember, "Progress, not perfection."

Food Prep for Thursday, Day 4

- ☐ Prepare and package snacks.
- ☐ Prepare 10-Layer Salad in a Jar with smoked turkey for lunch.
- ☐ Take a moment to regroup for the next three or four days. Look at the Meal Plan. What produce, refrigerator, and pantry items need to be replenished? Prepare a shopping list for the remainder of this week. Plan to go shopping tonight or tomorrow.

Day 4

Meal Plan

Breakfast	Snack (Optional)	Lunch	Snack (Required)	Dinner
Chocolate Cherry-Berry Smoothie (p. 230)	¼ cup Sweet Spiced Pepitas (p. 294)	10-Layer Salad in a Jar (p. 248) with organic deli-style smoked turkey and White Balsamic Vinaigrette (p. 286)	1 Pumpkin Spice Protein Bar (p. 241)	Lentil Soup (p. 260) and Dani's Mediterranean Chopped Salad (p. 282)

Inspiration

"The time has come to accept and embrace exactly who you are and exactly where you are today. Truly love yourself and realize deeply that you have great worth. Then decide and commit to heal past wounds, to do your best, and to improve yourself for yourself at your own pace every day from now on." —Doe Zantamata

Affirmation

"I am worthy of great things."

Diva Daily

Is there a PCOS symptom that is standing between you and the best version of yourself? For me it was hirsutism. Worrying about the hair growth on my chin took up much of the space in my head that could have been used for higher thoughts. It wasn't until I took charge of this symptom by researching and putting into action what I learned that I began to make progress. I discovered that laser hair removal worked wonders for me and eventually invested in an at-home laser. By combining that with the PCOS Diva lifestyle, I was able to greatly reduce this symptom, so it is no longer a worry. But it wouldn't have been possible if I hadn't researched to find solutions.

Diva Do

Knowledge is power. Action helps move you from victim to in control. PCOSDiva.com is a great place to begin your research. Take time today to visit the site and type a symptom that is bothering you in the search box. Is it hair loss, stress, fertility, anxiety? Read the available resources on these topics. Write the symptom down in your journal and record what you've learned. Start gathering additional information on the symptom and potential resolutions from trusted resources, and begin to take action to find a solution that works for you. With persistence and perseverance, you too can move beyond the struggle of PCOS to live the life you imagined.

Food Prep for Friday, Day 5

- ☐ Prepare and package snacks.
- ☐ Package planned-over Lentil Soup and mixed-greens salad for lunch.
- ☐ Wash, chop, and store veggies for snacks and salads for the next three days.

🌿 Day 5

Meal Plan

Breakfast	Snack (Optional)	Lunch	Snack (Required)	Dinner
1 Pumpkin Spice Protein Bar (p. 241)	⅓ cup shell-on pistachios	Planned-over Lentil Soup and mixed greens with White Balsamic Vinaigrette (p. 286)	⅓ cup Hummus (p. 292) and vegetable crudités	Maple-Mustard Salmon (p. 272), Whipped Butternut Squash (p. 278), and Garlicky Greens (p. 278)

Inspiration

"One of the marks of excellent people is that they never compare themselves with others. They only compare themselves with themselves and with their past accomplishments and future potential." —Brian Tracy

Affirmation

"I love taking good care of myself."

Diva Daily

You have begun to limit your screen time in the evening. Today, you will take this a step farther and begin to take charge of the media and messages you consume. Most media sell you the idea that you are not enough. You are only enough when you buy the ageless skin-care cream, perfect-body diet, or luxurious hair-care product or when you are the perfect mom and a superstar at your job. The more media you consume, the more you believe the story that you are not enough. Ads try to convince you that whatever they are selling is the missing piece to a perfect life. So much media today cultivates a feeling of lack and dis-ease.

Social media can be just as toxic. Looking at curated images of someone's life can drive even the most self-assured to think that their life is lacking. You can now can cover up pimples, whiten teeth, and air-brush with the swipe of a finger, creating images of perfection. People don't generally post that their kid got suspended from school or their relationship with their partner is on the rocks. You don't see the real, authentic, and sometimes messy lives, only the perfect stills.

As PCOS Divas, we must be very selective about the media we take in. Just as we feed our bodies nourishing food, we feed our minds nourishing media. Over time, I have crowded out much of my TV consumption and social-media scrolling with inspirational books, audiobooks, and podcasts.

I have a huge bookshelf containing books that further my understanding of nutrition and PCOS. Although these books are important, inspirational books provide a richness to my life and help me to repair the damage done from years of reading fashion magazines and comparing myself with what I saw on other people's Facebook pages.

"Comparison is the thief of joy."

—THEODORE ROOSEVELT

Early on, I realized that if I was going to live my life as a PCOS Diva, I had to upgrade my mindset. I found my first mindset mentors in books. The books that truly helped me grow were written by authors who had overcome adversity, especially those who shared actionable steps on how to improve the quality of my life. I also found it was important to feed my soul. Spiritually themed books satisfy my craving to live life on a deeper level. I always have a book or two on my nightstand or an audiobook on my phone.

I absolutely love audiobooks and podcasts. I listen while driving my kiddos around, grocery shopping, cooking dinner, and doing household chores. Right now I'm enjoying the Quote of the Day podcast by Sean Croxton. Each episode spotlights an inspiring quote and a 5- to 10-minute motivational audio clip.

Look for books and other media that feed your spirit and curiosity.

Diva Do

Spend 15 minutes today looking for a book that will uplift you. Sign up for an audiobook account or check out your local library. Libraries often have downloadable audiobooks as well. I promise, the more you make it a habit to read or listen to inspirational books, the more you crave them, and the more abundant your life will become.

Week Two Weekend Prep: Get a Running Start

Now is the time to begin planning and prep for Week Two. In addition to your daily food prep this weekend, you'll also do your weekend prep for next week.

- ☐ Look over the Week Two Meal Plan at a Glance (p. 160). Do you need to make any substitutions or rearrange the meals to fit your schedule? Using the Meal Plan and the meal-planning

—— A Few Inspirational Books to Get You Started ——

The Rhythm of Life, by Matthew Kelly

Begin with Yes, by Paul Boyton

Firestarter Sessions, by Danielle LaPorte

The Gifts of Imperfection, by Brené Brown

The War of Art, by Steven Pressfield

Honor Yourself, by Patricia Spadaro

Bonjour, Happiness! by Jamie Kat Callan

Beautiful You, by Rosie Molinary

---

tips in Step 9 of Chapter 6 (p. 108), plan your food for the week.

☐ Based upon your Meal Plan, make a detailed list of the grocery items you need for the week, from breakfasts through dinners, including snacks and replacement of staples. Look in your pantry and refrigerator. What do you have on hand and what do you need to put on your shopping list for the next four days?

☐ Grocery shop for the next three or four days.

☐ Prepare and package snacks for Week Two that can be made in advance, for example, 5-Layer Trail Mix (p. 294).

☐ Wash, chop, and store veggies for snacks and salads for the first three or four days.

☐ Make a batch or two of Terrific Tahini Dressing (p. 287).

Food Prep for Saturday, Day 6

☐ Prepare and package snacks.

☐ Prepare 10-Layer Salad in a Jar with salmon for lunch.

☐ Plan where you will go out to dinner. Review online menus to determine whether the offerings will fit into the Healing PCOS Plan (see Tips for Dining Out, p. 63).

☐ Prepare Overnight Blueberry Buckle Steel-Cut Oats to cook overnight in the slow cooker. Or prepare the ingredients to make it in a rice cooker or on the stovetop in the morning.

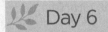 Day 6

Meal Plan

Breakfast	Snack (Optional)	Lunch	Snack (Required)	Dinner
Overnight Blueberry Buckle Steel-Cut Oats (p. 238)	1 small sliced pear with 2 tablespoons sunflower-seed butter, sprinkled with hemp or chia seeds	10-Layer Salad in a Jar (p. 248) with salmon and White Balsamic Vinaigrette (p. 286)	1 hard-boiled egg and vegetable crudités	EAT OUT

Inspiration

"The soul becomes dyed with the color of its thoughts."
—Marcus Aurelius

Affirmation

"I am changing my habits by changing my thoughts."

Diva Daily

Switching your viewpoint of life from one of scarcity or lack to one of abundance can completely change your life. The first step is awareness.

Diva Do

Today you will take inventory of your dominant thoughts. Use your journal to help you with this activity. Every time you catch yourself coming from a place of scarcity or lack, write it down in your journal. For example:

"I'm afraid I won't have enough money to pay my bills at the end of the month."

"It's not fair that I have PCOS and can't eat whatever I want."

"I wish I looked like Cindy. She is so tall and glamorous."

"Why can't I have a beautiful life like Jacquie? She has it all—great job, great husband, lots of vacations."

"I never have enough time to make healthy meals."

Refer to p. 41 for a list of Lack Thinking examples. See how many of these you encounter during your day today and write them down.

Once you start noticing these scarcity or lack thoughts, you can begin to deliberately turn them around. At the end of the day today, reframe these thoughts from the perspective of abundance. For example:

"I will never lose weight" becomes "I will find a balanced weight."

"I never have time to exercise" becomes "I love the way my body feels when I move it, and I will find the time."

"I'll never look pretty" becomes "I exude a healthy radiance."

"I never have enough money" becomes "I have enough money to cover what I truly need."

At first you may feel as though you are lying to yourself, but even if you don't believe the reframed thoughts, the trick is to step into positivity, appreciation, and gratitude. Focus, feel grateful, and appreciate what you do have. Hold this feeling as often as you can, especially when worry or fear enters your mind.

Think of it this way. One road in life is paved with scarcity and the other with abundance. At every turn, at every moment, you get to choose which road you want to travel. You can have joy every day of your life. It is all about your mindset.

Food Prep for Sunday, Day 7

☐ Prepare and package snacks.
☐ Prepare 10-Layer Salad in a Jar with smoked turkey for lunch.

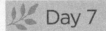 Day 7

Meal Plan

Breakfast	Snack (Optional)	Lunch	Snack (Required)	Dinner
Lemon Poppy-Seed Pancakes (p. 245)	¼ cup Sweet Spiced Pepitas (p. 294)	10-Layer Salad in a Jar (p. 248) with organic deli-style smoked turkey and White Balsamic Vinaigrette (p. 286)	celery sticks and 2 tablespoons cashew butter with 5 dried cranberries	Grass-fed sirloin steak with Chimichurri Sauce (p. 288), Grilled Cauliflower Steaks with Sweet Vidalia Onions (p. 281), and foil-packet sweet potatoes (4-Step Grilled Veggies, p. 280)

Inspiration

"The flower doesn't dream of the bee. It blossoms, and the bee comes."
—Mark Nepo

Affirmation

"I am creating healthy habits that support my goals."

Diva Daily

Discovering your PCOS Diva is about becoming more mindful. You've become more mindful and present about the way you go about your day, instituting new habits and rituals. You've also become more mindful about the way you think, the food you eat, and how it makes you feel. Now you will learn to eat mindfully.

Express gratitude. Begin your meal with gratitude, whether you offer a prayer of thanksgiving or simply bring to mind all of the people whose effort it took to put this food on your table, from farmers to pickers, to truck drivers and grocery-store workers.

Pause. Take a moment before you begin to eat to notice and appreciate the food's texture, visual appeal, and aroma. This brief pause helps you to become more present before you begin eating.

Eat mindfully. Turn off the TV, phone, computer, or any other distraction. Sit down. Don't eat standing up at the counter or while driving the car. Focus on the utensils and act of putting the food in your mouth. Then be mindful of the flavor and texture while you chew. Focus on chewing a bit longer than you normally would (shoot for twenty times). Try to put down your utensil between bites. From time to time, take a moment to draw a mindful breath or even a sip of water.

Acknowledge. Thoughts, feelings, and sensations will arise as you are eating. Don't push them away. Acknowledge them and then let them pass by, like a cloud that floats overhead. Then return to eating mindfully.

Diva Do

Today, do two things.

Commit to eating mindfully during at least one meal every day for the rest of the program.

Look at the data you've collected in your journal on your physical and emotional responses to food. Do you notice any patterns? Are there any theories you'd like to test next week? Maybe you are beginning to realize that unhealthy food isn't as delicious as you thought or that it doesn't make you feel very good. Perhaps you are beginning to see how food affects your mood and energy level throughout the day. You might be discovering which foods give you the most vitality for your exercise, work, and leisure. Do you feel as though you need the morning snack? Are you starving by dinner? Did you feel you needed a nap after having the Lentil Soup lunch? Do you crave the office donuts when you have a smoothie for breakfast but not when you have a protein bar? Look through your journal and note your observations.

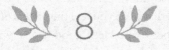

8

Week Two:

LIVE

Changing your habits and lifestyle isn't easy. It takes determination, persistence, patience, and perseverance. I hope you are learning that it doesn't require perfection. Perhaps the most important elements to create sustainable positive change are kindness, grace, and forgiveness *toward yourself.*

You may have begun to worry about how long you'll be able to stick with the plan, rationalizing that you've never been able to follow any diet long-term. It is important to remind yourself to take it one day at a time, one step at a time, one moment at a time. When it becomes clear that a day isn't unfolding as planned, be gentle, extend yourself some grace, and make the next best choice to move forward.

Don't allow negative self-talk. If you find yourself thinking, "I can't do this. I'll always be overweight, infertile, tired, _____ (fill in the blank). I'm not enough," immediately flip the script. Tell your-self—out loud—"I CAN do this; it just takes time and practice. I don't have to learn everything at once." Negative self-talk usually stems from disappointing past experiences with quick-fix diets based on depriva-tion and denial. Remember that the Healing PCOS Plan is not a fad diet. It is a nourishing and nurturing lifestyle. The key difference is that it is a *sustainable* way of living. Since PCOS must be managed over the course of a lifetime, you must learn new ways of thinking, moving, and eating in order to thrive. This takes time. Be patient and kind to yourself. You'll find that once you feel the effects of your good choices, you will get into a positive cycle: a good choice will leave you feeling good, so you make another good choice, and so on. You will find the momentum to move forward and continue to *live like a PCOS Diva for a lifetime.*

By now you should be feeling some of the rewards of the Healing PCOS Plan—brighter eyes, clearer thinking, more energy, and a more optimistic mood. Let this propel you forward through Week Two, Live Week.

During Week Two, you will reinforce the habits created during Week One and follow the same daily protocol. In addition, we will explore ways to create a movement mindset and look for ways to add more movement to your day. Movement is essential to help lower stress levels, improve mood, and lift anxiety and worry.

Hopefully, you've been walking for 15 minutes after lunch or dinner (or both) as part of the daily routine you established in Week One. How will you add more movement? As a start, you will get up 15 minutes earlier to create space in your daily routine to add Morning Movement. I like to do sun salutations and then jump on my rebounder for a few minutes to get the blood pumping.

In addition, you are going to find some time for Bonus Movement each day. You will either add HIIT to your daily walk(s), add 10 minutes of strength training, or add 10 minutes of a mind–body exercise:

HIIT: Add intervals to your daily walk(s). For example:

3-minute warmup: Walk at a leisurely pace to help prepare your joints, muscles, and heart for exercise.

1-minute power walk: Walk at a brisk pace; it should be hard to carry on a conversation.

2-minute recovery: Reduce speed to a moderate pace, but one that is somewhat faster than warmup.

1-minute power walk: Walk at a brisk pace.

2-minute recovery: Reduce speed to a moderate pace.

1-minute power walk: Walk at a brisk pace.

2-minute recovery: Reduce speed to a moderate pace.

3-minute cooldown: Cool down at a leisurely pace.

Strength training: Find a 10-minute body weight routine online. A quick search will yield dozens of free workout ideas. Commit to doing it two to three times this week. Slot this into your calendar as self-care time.

Mind–body movement: Do a 10-minute series of sun salutations or simple stretches. There are countless routines available on YouTube and Pinterest. Take a moment to find one that you will practice this week. Plan at least one series in your calendar as self-care time this week.

Week Two Meal Plan at a Glance

Monday, Day 8

Breakfast	Snack (Optional)	Lunch	Snack (Required)	Dinner
Sausage, Asparagus, and Egg Muffin Cups (p. 240)	½ cup fresh or frozen berries and ¼ cup almonds	10-Layer Salad in a Jar (p. 248) with steak and Terrific Tahini Dressing (p. 287)	¼ cup Sweet Spiced Pepitas (p. 294)	Sesame-Crusted Chicken Strips (p. 270) with Spicy Raspberry Dipping Sauce (p. 290), ½ medium roasted butternut squash (6-Step Roasted Veggies, p. 275), and Orange Fennel Slaw (p. 283)

Tuesday, Day 9

Breakfast	Snack (Optional)	Lunch	Snack (Required)	Dinner
Chocolate-Almond-Strawberry Chia Pudding (p. 233)	1 Pumpkin Spice Protein Bar (p. 241)	10-Layer Salad in a Jar (p. 248) with chicken and Terrific Tahini Dressing (p. 287)	1 small sliced apple with 2 tablespoons sunflower-seed butter, sprinkled with hemp or chia seeds	White Chicken Chili (p. 256) and mixed greens with Avocado-Lime Ranch Dressing (p. 287)

Wednesday, Day 10

Breakfast	Snack (Optional)	Lunch	Snack (Required)	Dinner
Apple Cobbler Super-Seed Quick Oats (p. 236)	¼ cup 5-Layer Trail Mix (p. 294)	Planned-over White Chicken Chili and mixed greens with Avocado-Lime Ranch Dressing (p. 287)	6 Mary's Gone Crackers and ⅓ cup Rosemary White Bean Dip (p. 292)	Caribbean Salmon and Pineapple Kabobs (p. 274), Quinoa Pilaf (p. 279), and mixed greens with Terrific Tahini Dressing (p. 287)

Thursday, Day 11

Breakfast	Snack (Optional)	Lunch	Snack (Required)	Dinner
Ginger Peach Smoothie (p. 230)	¼ cup Sweet Spiced Pepitas (p. 294)	10-Layer Salad in a Jar (p. 248) with salmon and Terrific Tahini Dressing (p. 287)	1 Pumpkin Spice Protein Bar (p. 241)	Spring Greens Soup (p. 261), Lemon-Pepper Chicken Drumsticks (p. 271), and vegetable crudités with Avocado-Lime Ranch Dressing (p. 287)

Friday, Day 12

Breakfast	Snack (Optional)	Lunch	Snack (Required)	Dinner
Spinach, Tomato, and Basil Egg Scramble (p. 239)	¼ cup 5-Layer Trail Mix (p. 294)	Planned-over Spring Greens Soup and Lemon-Pepper Chicken Drumsticks	6 Mary's Gone Crackers and ⅓ cup Rosemary White Bean Dip (p. 292)	Citrus Fajitas (p. 268) with Cashew-Lime Crema (p. 290) and broccoli with Lemon-Dijon Sauce (p. 291)

Saturday, Day 13

Breakfast	Snack (Optional)	Lunch	Snack (Required)	Dinner
Apple Pie Smoothie (p. 229)	celery sticks and 2 tablespoons cashew butter with 5 dried cranberries	10-Layer Salad in a Jar (p. 248) with planned-over Citrus Fajitas, guacamole, and salsa	¼ cup 5-Layer Trail Mix (p. 294)	EAT OUT

Sunday, Day 14

Breakfast	Snack (Optional)	Lunch	Snack (Required)	Dinner
Fruit Scone (p. 243)	¼ cup 5-Layer Trail Mix (p. 294)	Layered Lunch Wrap (p. 252) with Curried Egg Salad (p. 252)	½ cup fresh or frozen berries and ¼ cup almonds	Savory Salisbury Steak (p. 262), Root Veggie Mash (p. 279), roasted asparagus (6-Step Roasted Veggies, p. 275), and sliced tomato

Live: Week Two Daily Protocol

☐ Bonus Movement: HIIT added to walk(s), 10 minutes of strength training, or 10 minutes of mind–body exercise sometime during the day

Rocket Launch. *Wake up 15 minutes earlier than usual.*
  ☐ Morning Motto
  ☐ Big Why
  ☐ Gratitude

Morning Reflection
  ☐ Morning elixir
  ☐ Inspiration

- ☐ Affirmation
- ☐ 15-minute Morning Movement

Shower
- ☐ Dry brushing before shower
- ☐ Oil massage after shower

Breakfast
- ☐ Meal
- ☐ Breakfast supplements
- ☐ Tongue scrape

Daily Lesson
- ☐ Diva Daily
- ☐ Diva Do
- ☐ Movement Mindset

Morning Snack/Tea Time
- ☐ Optional snack
- ☐ Beverage break

Lunch
- ☐ Meal
- ☐ Lunch supplements
- ☐ 15-minute walk

Afternoon Snack/Tea Time
- ☐ Required snack
- ☐ Beverage break
- ☐ Water check (have you had enough water today?)

Dinner
- ☐ Meal
- ☐ Dinner supplements
- ☐ 15-minute walk
- ☐ Dessert chocolate (optional)
- ☐ Next day food prep

Nighttime Ritual
- ☐ Unplugged by 8 p.m.
- ☐ Evening elixir and/or evening snack (only if needed)
- ☐ Tomorrow's Priority List

- ☐ Magnesium
- ☐ Tongue scrape
- ☐ Essential oils
- ☐ Stretching
- ☐ Book
- ☐ Gratitude stone
- ☐ Sleep mask and lights out by 10 p.m.

Food Prep for Monday, Day 8

- ☐ Prepare and package snacks.
- ☐ Prepare 10-Layer Salad in a Jar with steak for lunch.
- ☐ Peel and chop ½ medium butternut squash into 1-inch pieces. Place in the refrigerator for tomorrow. Review 6-Step Roasted Veggies for flavor layering (coconut oil, Pumpkin Pie Spice, or maple syrup drizzle works well) and cooking directions.
- ☐ Chop the fennel bulb and 1 cup red cabbage and refrigerate for Orange Fennel Slaw.
- ☐ Prepare and bake Sausage, Asparagus, and Egg Muffin Cups if you will be short on time in the morning. Store two in the refrigerator for breakfast. Freeze the remaining muffin cups for future.

🌿 Day 8

Meal Plan

Breakfast	Snack (Optional)	Lunch	Snack (Required)	Dinner
Sausage, Asparagus, and Egg Muffin Cups (p. 240)	½ cup fresh or frozen berries and ¼ cup almonds	10-Layer Salad in a Jar (p. 248) with steak and Terrific Tahini Dressing (p. 287)	¼ cup Sweet Spiced Pepitas (p. 294)	Sesame-Crusted Chicken Strips (p. 270) with Spicy Raspberry Dipping Sauce (p. 290), ½ medium roasted butternut squash (6-Step Roasted Veggies, p. 275), and Orange Fennel Slaw (p. 283)

Inspiration

"All healing starts with beginning to accept yourself and love yourself, even your flaws." —Bryant McGill

Affirmation

"I am healthy and radiant."

Diva Daily

I achieved my Weight Watcher lifetime-member status in my mid-twenties, but to be honest, the Weight Watcher point mentality and my perfectionist tendencies just didn't mix. If I messed up and went over my points before the week was over, I would beat myself up and tell myself I'd start fresh on Monday, even if it was Wednesday. Then I'd let things go until, in my mind, I had a clean slate again on Monday and would start the cycle all over again. The Healing PCOS 21-Day Plan is deliberately different. There are no metrics, carbs to count, or points to accrue. If you get off track or make a mistake, *you are always, always, one choice away from getting back on track.*

Everyone messes up. We are not perfect. We all do things we don't consciously mean to do. The critical concept for you to take away is to be kind to yourself and forgive yourself. You deserve forgiveness. You would certainly forgive your child, so why not yourself?

Rather than feeling guilt or shame, see it as an opportunity to grow. Although it is important to acknowledge mistakes and learn from them, it is equally important to let yourself off the hook. If something didn't go as well as you liked last week, think about how you can better prepare and create space for success. Maybe you need to make sure you have snacks in the car, or put your robe and slippers by the bed the night before so you feel cozier as soon as you rocket-launch. How can you better plan for success?

Diva Do

Reflect on Discover Week. When I coach clients, most answer the question "How did your week go?" by telling me about all of the things that didn't go well. Rather than dwelling on what hasn't been working, acknowledge what *is* working. What went well over the last week? What were your wins? Or, as I like to start my coaching sessions, "What's new and good?" Write down the answers in your journal.

Now focus on the week ahead. Think about how amazing you can make it. Reflect upon your Big Why and write down three goals for your week.

Movement Mindset

Exercise has many physical benefits including weight loss, improved metabolic markers, and increased fertility, but it may take weeks or months to see these results. Rather than concentrating solely on physical benefits, focus on how movement helps to change your mood. When I'm in a rotten mood, my husband reminds me to go to the gym or take a walk. Sometimes he literally has to hand me the keys and put me in the car or hand me my shoes and push me out the door. But he is right; after moving for 10 minutes, I feel a mood boost.

Tune into your mental state before and after you move today. Rate how you feel on a scale of 1 to 10 before moving and rate how you feel again after. Allow this improvement (and I promise you, your mood will improve) to create sustainability.

Food Prep for Tuesday, Day 9

☐ Prepare and package snacks.

☐ Prepare Chocolate-Almond-Strawberry Chia Pudding and place in the refrigerator for breakfast.

☐ Prepare 10-Layer Salad in a Jar with chicken for lunch.

☐ Cook chicken for White Chicken Chili.

☐ Prepare Avocado-Lime Ranch Dressing.

🌿 Day 9

Meal Plan

Breakfast	Snack (Optional)	Lunch	Snack (Required)	Dinner
Chocolate-Almond-Strawberry Chia Pudding (p. 233)	1 Pumpkin Spice Protein Bar (p. 241)	10-Layer Salad in a Jar (p. 248) with chicken and Terrific Tahini Dressing (p. 287)	1 small sliced apple with 2 tablespoons sunflower-seed butter, sprinkled with hemp or chia seeds	White Chicken Chili (p. 256) and mixed greens with Avocado-Lime Ranch Dressing (p. 287)

Inspiration

"Be there for others, but never leave yourself behind." —Dodinsky

Affirmation

"I deserve to take care of myself."

Diva Daily

I've learned that when I am crabby, irritable, and feeling burned out, it is a sign that I need to find time for more "sweet stuff" in my life.

Similarly, when I find myself craving sugar and I know it isn't because of a physical blood-sugar imbalance, then I know I need more "sweet stuff."

Many of us struggle with using food to fill a hunger we have in another part of our lives. We need nourishment in many forms. We all have a real need for love, friendship, laughter, movement, creativity, purpose, spirituality, meaningful work, relaxation, and beauty. We must feed our whole being, or we will end up full of food but never really satisfied.

Now instead of automatically reaching for something sweet when a craving hits, I ask myself, "What am I really hungry for?" Typically, I can find the answer on my Sweet Stuff list, an emergency go-to list of all the things that make me happy, fulfilled, joyful, and recharged. The things on my list provide ways for me to find sweetness and nourishment in nonfood ways.

I try to schedule something from my Sweet Stuff list on my calendar every day. Of course, the day doesn't always go as I planned, especially

---

Amy's Sweet Stuff

Not only has this list helped me kick a sugar habit, it has helped me feel happier and more peaceful, grounded, and balanced.

- Taking a detox bath.
- Taking a 30-minute nap.
- Coloring with my daughter.
- Shooting hoops with my boys.
- Going on a date with my husband.
- Having coffee with a friend.
- Visiting the farmers' market.
- Going for an acupuncture treatment.
- Setting the timer for 15 minutes and decluttering a drawer or closet.
- Paying it forward and buying coffee for the person behind me at the drive-thru.

---

with three kids, but it is still a step in the right direction to at least include myself on my schedule.

I've come to realize that self-care is nonnegotiable if I want to live life as a PCOS Diva. I know that not taking care of myself in this way only sets me up to eventually explode in an emotional tirade of yelling and tears. I am a better wife, mother, and friend when I take care of myself. *The more I give to me, the more I have to give to others.*

Diva Do

Create your own Sweet Stuff list and then schedule three items from the list on your calendar this week. Try not to save your Sweet Stuff (unless it is a relaxing bath) for the end of the day when you are too tired to move and your brain has stopped working. Take care of yourself first; if necessary, take a break during your day. This time is not a reward for good behavior and should not be contingent on doing anything "right." Self-care is an important element of thriving as a PCOS Diva.

Movement Mindset

Find your Big Why for moving your body. If your Big Why is to look more attractive in order to please others, dig deeper.

Through my teens and twenties, my motivation to work out was to reduce the size of what I thought was my big butt. As a junior in high school, I had overheard a seventeen-year-old boy say, "She'd be cute if it wasn't for her big butt." This boy influenced my Big Why for the next decade. I would run for miles on the treadmill or road trying to literally run my butt off. It took all of the joy out of exercising. I finally came to embrace my round derriere. Enhancing what God has given me actually became one of the reasons I love barre workouts. Many of the movements are meant to lift and tone what the instructors refer to as your "seat."

But my Big Why for moving is no longer to look good in a bathing suit, but rather to give me the energy and the grounded, stable, and uplifted mood to be the best version of myself I can be, for myself, my family, and to do the work of PCOS Diva. This Big Why creates a more sustainable and joy-filled *movement mindset.*

Take some time today to consider why movement should be a part of your life. To increase your fertility? To be able to play tag with your kids without feeling like you are going pass out? To feel strong? Write down your Big Why to keep you moving forward.

Food Prep for Wednesday, Day 10

☐ Make Rosemary White Bean Dip.
☐ Prepare and package snacks.
☐ Package planned-over White Chicken Chili and mixed-greens salad for lunch.

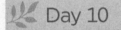 Day 10

Meal Plan

Breakfast	Snack (Optional)	Lunch	Snack (Required)	Dinner
Apple Cobbler Super-Seed Quick Oats (p. 236)	¼ cup 5-Layer Trail Mix (p. 294)	Planned-over White Chicken Chili and mixed greens with Avocado-Lime Ranch Dressing (p. 287)	6 Mary's Gone Crackers and ⅓ cup Rosemary White Bean Dip (p. 292)	Caribbean Salmon and Pineapple Kabobs (p. 274), Quinoa Pilaf (p. 279), and mixed greens with Terrific Tahini Dressing (p. 287)

Inspiration

"When you can't change the direction of the wind—adjust your sails."
—H. Jackson Brown, Jr.

Affirmation

"I am stronger than my negative thoughts."

Diva Daily

When you have PCOS, it can be easy to dwell on what you feel you are not: not fertile enough, not feminine enough, not thin enough. Just plain not enough. We often spend our mental energy focusing on what is wrong with us, but I want you to realize that you are more than what you lack. Once you shift from dwelling on what you are *not* to celebrating what you *are*, then you can begin to truly heal.

Celebrating who you are, what makes you unique, your strengths and gifts begins with awareness. It was hard for me to put a finger on what my gifts were. I was so focused on all of the things I lacked that I really didn't know what made me special. I needed to realize what I brought to this world and begin using those gifts. Once I began this process, my life became much more joy-filled. Sure, PCOS is part of who you are, and if you can come to a place of acceptance (and as we will explore in Chapter 10, even gratitude), the journey will become easier.

Diva Do

Three tools helped me to discover my own unique character traits and strengths. The first is the Jung Typology Test, a free personality test created by Humanmetrics and based on Carl Jung's and Isabel Briggs Myers's personality-type theories. (Please note that this is not the official Myers-Briggs Type Indicator personality test that is administered by certified MBTI practitioners. For more information on the MBTI, see http://www.myersbriggs.org/my-mbti-personality-type/.)

I am an INFJ. When I started learning more about my INFJ personality traits, I discovered that this personality type is very rare, making up less than 1 percent of the population. I always thought that my traits and talents were the same as everyone else's and that we just applied them differently. They are actually unique gifts. I took my strengths for granted. I've since learned to celebrate all of the things that I am: creative, insightful, inspiring, decisive, determined, passionate, and altruistic. Take the test and see what you learn about yourself.

I also like the VIA Survey of Character Strengths. It is a free, simple self-assessment that takes less than 15 minutes and provides a wealth of information to help you understand your core characteristics. It was created under the direction of Dr. Martin Seligman, the "father of positive psychology" and author of *Authentic Happiness* and *Flourish*. My top three character strengths are love of learning, social intelligence, and spirituality.

When I'm using my gifts, writing this book, for instance, I'm in a state of flow. Time sort of goes away. It seems as if it has only been 15 minutes, and when I look up, it has been three hours. As the mythologist Joseph Campbell would say, I am following my bliss. When I use my strengths, I feel happy, have less stress and more vitality, and am more content with my life. If you do the same, you will be too.

Finally, I love the "How to Fascinate" personality test created by Sally Hogshead. This test measures how others perceive you at your best as a way of identifying your unique strengths and gifts. After you answer twenty-eight short questions, the test reveals your hidden talents and personality archetype. As the website says, "The best parts of you might not have been obvious to you before. But now they can be." I have done this test with all of the members of my family, and it is really uncanny how accurate the results are. It reaffirmed what I already considered to be their gifts and helped them to see them for themselves. According to How to Fascinate, I'm a "wise owl": observant, assured, unruffled, logical, and nuanced. I'm watchful of the details and systematically approach problems to find the best solutions. It feels good to know what makes me unique, and this knowledge helps me to capitalize on my strengths and gifts.

I suggest that you:

1. Take the Jung Typology Test (www.humanmetrics.com) and then learn more about your type on the 16 Personalities website (www.16personalities.com).
2. Take the VIA Survey of Character Strengths (www.viacharacter.org).
3. Take the How to Fascinate Personality Test (www.howtofascinate.com).
4. Then take time today to recognize and celebrate your unique talents.

Movement Mindset

What is holding you back from getting out there and moving your body in ways that feel good? For a lot of women, it is the fear of being seen and judged. My client Vicky told me that she loved to swim. When I asked her why she didn't swim regularly, I thought she would say that she just didn't have access to a swimming pool, but instead she said, "I'd have to put on a bathing suit!" Well, yes that is true. It turned out that Vicky didn't want to put on a bathing suit, because she thought that everyone at the YMCA pool would stare at her and judge her. As an outsider, it was easy for me to see that her fear of being seen and judged was a self-limiting belief that was acting as barrier to what she wanted.

Today, identify your limiting beliefs in connection with movement. The longer we hold on to a belief, the more it becomes ingrained in our minds; it seems like it is "truth" when in fact it is not. It may take a friend or spouse to help you uncover your limiting beliefs.

Make a list of your limiting beliefs connected with movement. What limiting beliefs are keeping you from moving your body in ways that you love and that feel good? Is it that you think people will judge you? Or you might get injured? Or you just don't have the time or money? Write them all down in your journal.

How have these limiting beliefs kept you from experiencing the fullness and joy of life? Vicky realized that her limiting belief was holding her back from doing what she loved and fueling a sense of lack, that she was not enough.

About each belief, ask yourself the following three questions:

1. Where does this belief come from?
2. What evidence do I have that the belief is true? What real circumstances have happened in the last year that support any truth in my limiting belief?
3. Could this belief be sort of ridiculous if I looked at it as an outsider?

You may have to enlist a partner or friend to help you with number 3. Often you can have a laugh about how crazy the limiting belief is when you look at it from the outside. Other times, it is a mindset issue that will take time and perseverance to overcome.

Neutralize the limiting belief with positive visualization. Visualize a positive outcome. Vicky visualized herself heading to the pool with her head held high, shoulders back, and a smile on her face, thinking all the way how good it would feel to be in the water swimming. Spend a few minutes visualizing your positive outcome.

After going through this exercise, Vicky was able to move beyond her limiting belief. Instead of dwelling on what was holding her back from moving her body in ways that she loved and that felt good, she focused on her Big Why, which was getting healthy, so she could be a better mom for her son. She realized that what she once thought was a truth was just a mirage. She realized that without dwelling on the negative limiting belief, she was free to live her life on her terms. She was free to live abundantly. She was free to do what was important to her. Imagine what you can accomplish and how great you will feel when you have dispelled your limiting beliefs.

Food Prep for Thursday, Day 11

- ☐ Prepare and package snacks.
- ☐ Prepare 10-Layer Salad in a Jar with salmon for lunch.
- ☐ Marinate Lemon-Pepper Chicken Drumsticks overnight.
- ☐ Take a moment to look ahead to the next three or four days. Look at the Meal Plan. What produce, refrigerator, and pantry items need to be replenished? Prepare a shopping list for the remainder of this week. Plan to go shopping tonight or tomorrow.

Day 11

Meal Plan

Breakfast	Snack (Optional)	Lunch	Snack (Required)	Dinner
Ginger Peach Smoothie (p. 230)	¼ cup Sweet Spiced Pepitas (p. 294)	10-Layer Salad in a Jar (p. 248) with salmon and Terrific Tahini Dressing (p. 287)	1 Pumpkin Spice Protein Bar (p. 241)	Spring Greens Soup (p. 261), Lemon-Pepper Chicken Drumsticks (p. 271), and vegetable crudités with Avocado-Lime Ranch Dressing (p. 287)

Inspiration

"One day she finally grasped that unexpected things were always going to happen in life. And with that she realized the only control she had was how she chose to handle them. So, she made the decision to survive using courage, humor, and grace. She was the Queen of her own life and the choice was hers." —Kathy Kinney, Queenofyourownlife.com

Affirmation

"I am allowed to say no to others and yes to myself."

Diva Daily

For many of us, deciding to say no to others is a constant battle. By declining a request, we worry that we will be perceived as impolite or selfish. But as difficult as it may be, it is essential to your well-being to say no when you want or need to. It's okay to appear selfish when it comes to your health.

It is hard to say no, especially if we are people pleasers and fear disappointing or hurting someone. So we often say yes to others at the expense of ourselves. We can spend way too much time and energy trying to keep others happy. Yet we are not responsible for anyone else's reaction, and it is far better to feel uncomfortable saying no than resentful saying yes. In order to thrive, we must create space in our lives dedicated to self-care, enjoyment, and pleasure. Yet our lives are often filled with so many obligations and mandatory commitments that it's hard to squeeze in "me time" for rest and recovery.

If I don't squeeze in this time, I end up frustrated and stressed, and I don't have the space to say yes to the really important things. I find it helpful to think of my wellness and happiness on a spectrum; the more I commit to things I prefer not to, the farther I move away from my vision of living like a PCOS Diva. I love this sentiment by one of my favorite authors, Katrina Kenison, as it sums up this idea perfectly: "Solitude is the soul's holiday, an opportunity to stop doing for others and to surprise and delight ourselves instead."

Diva Do

Today say yes to the things that make your soul feel happy. Say yes to the things that give you enjoyment, that benefit you, that contribute positively to your health or add meaning to your life. Life is too full of things that we can't choose to say yes or no to—so we need to make all of our other time count. Start spending more time saying yes to yourself and less time regretting decisions. Setting boundaries is not only empowering; it's necessary to your health, your progress, and channeling your energy into what truly matters to you.

Movement Mindset

Any form of movement done as a means of "beating yourself up" is harmful. Exercising out of compulsion, excessive competition, or lack of self-acceptance is a sign of a dis-eased, unbalanced movement mindset. It doesn't matter if the exercise is yoga, running, or dancing.

I used to run to punish myself for having a body that didn't co-operate with me, for having a body that had more fat than I wanted. I didn't run because I loved movement. Now on a warm summer day I love to go for a run. It brings me joy and nourishes me, because I give myself permission to do it in a way that feels good. I allow myself to go slower and add walk breaks. I listen to joyful music and am very mindful of the beauty of nature. Instead of focusing on my pace, beating my previous time, or how many calories I've burned, I focus on the entire sensory experience and all of the things I am grateful for. Those feelings of happiness and gratitude propel me forward. It is a completely different movement experience than running on a treadmill to burn calories.

When was the last time you exercised and felt better, mentally and physically, than before you began? When was the last time you felt balanced, nourished, and happy after moving your body? It is okay if the last time was when you were a child. Try to recall what you were doing. Whatever it is, bring more of that kind of movement into your life. Maybe what you loved to do falls within the categories of HIIT, strength training, or mind–body exercise. If it does, wonderful. But even if it doesn't, don't let that keep you from moving. Begin shifting your mindset to realize that movement isn't just a chore you do a few times a week. Movement is a lifestyle in which you move as much as possible because it feels good.

Food Prep for Friday, Day 12

- ☐ Prepare and package snacks.
- ☐ Package planned-over Spring Greens Soup and Lemon-Pepper Chicken Drumsticks for lunch.
- ☐ Marinate chicken or steak for Citrus Fajitas overnight.
- ☐ Soak cashews for Cashew-Lime Crema overnight.
- ☐ Wash, chop, and store veggies for snacks and salads for the next three days.

🌿 Day 12

Meal Plan

Breakfast	Snack (Optional)	Lunch	Snack (Required)	Dinner
Spinach, Tomato, and Basil Egg Scramble (p. 239)	¼ cup 5-Layer Trail Mix (p. 294)	Planned-over Spring Greens Soup and Lemon-Pepper Chicken Drumsticks	6 Mary's Gone Crackers and ⅓ cup Rosemary White Bean Dip (p. 292)	Citrus Fajitas (p. 268) with Cashew-Lime Crema (p. 290) and broccoli with Lemon-Dijon Sauce (p. 291)

Inspiration

"Even the smallest changes in our daily routine can create incredible ripple effects that expand our vision of what is possible."
—Charles F. Glassman

Affirmation

"Abundance flows into my life with ease."

Diva Daily

The simple ritual of afternoon tea—selecting, brewing, sipping, and savoring a cup of tea—can elevate you above the chaos of life. The stolen moment with a cup of tea allows for a pause in a hectic day, provides an opportunity to be mindful of blessings, and fortifies you, so you can take on the remainder of your day a bit more energized, centered, and balanced.

In addition to all of the health benefits of tea discussed in Chapter 4, research shows that even brief periods of relaxation can reduce cortisol levels, lower heart rates, and make us feel less anxious and stressed. A double-blind study in which half of the subjects incorporated tea into their lives for six weeks found that those drinking tea had significantly lower cortisol levels and a greater sense of relaxation.

Daily Do

Hopefully, you have been enjoying a cup of hot tea during afternoon snack time as laid out in the plan. Today step up this habit to create a tea ritual of sorts for yourself. You will prepare, sip, and savor your tea in a very mindful way, much like the way you've been eating your chocolate. Think of your afternoon teatime as an opportunity for extreme self-care and stress reduction. If you have an heirloom tea service in a china cabinet or in a box in your attic, now is the time to get it out of storage and put it to good use. If you don't have a pretty little teapot and special cup, make a point to treat yourself and purchase one in the near future. If you work in an office, think about investing in a stash of your own tea and a tea ball infuser. Bring your favorite cup to work to use.

Relaxation begins with choosing the tea. Check in with yourself. What kind of tea will hit the spot today? Perhaps a refreshing spearmint, hearty spiced black chai, a flowery oolong, or astringent matcha?

I've become somewhat of a tea snob. Gone are the days of grabbing a box of grocery-store tea bags. Although conventional tea bags are convenient, commercially produced tea is harvested with machines that take both old and new leaves as well as twigs from the plants. Another problem with commercially produced bagged tea is that the tea bags are bleached with chlorine, which can leach into the tea during steeping. The chlorine also contributes to the shorter shelf life of tea-bag tea, approximately six months. Loose-leaf tea, if stored properly, can last up to a year and a half.

With most loose-leaf tea, only the top two leaves and bud are hand plucked and used. These young parts contain the most antioxidants; the longer the leaves spend on the bush, the fewer the health benefits. There is something extra special about opening a tin of loose-leaf tea, inhaling the fragrance of the leaves, and spooning it into a pretty teapot. Experiment with different teas. See how they make your body feel, and find ones that suit both your tastes and your moods. I love a cup of matcha in the morning, Earl Grey in the afternoon, and chamomile before bedtime.

Spoon out the tea leaves, 1 teaspoon per cup.

Add water to a kettle and set it over heat. If you are really being per-snickety, you'll want the water between 165 and 195 degrees F., which is below boiling. You don't want to burn the tea leaves.

When the water is ready, *pour the water over the tea as if you're watering a plant,* and let the tea steep for 3 to 5 minutes. The tea becomes more bitter the longer it brews.

The most powerful part of the ritual is patience. You must wait for the water to rise to the right temperature. You must wait to let the tea leaves steep. You can't rush the process. It will take the time that it will take. These are the mindful moments that ground me during my day. I don't try to fit in another email or unload the dishwasher. I take these moments just for me. I gaze out the window and notice a blooming flower or busy bee. I think of the blessings of the day. I breathe in the aroma of the tea.

Sip the tea slowly, savoring the warm, full flavor. You can't drink a cup of hot tea quickly, so give yourself permission to slow down and take these few moments just for you. It is a sweet surrender. I promise you'll finish your cup with a renewed sense of calm and peace.

Movement Mindset

When I was in my late teens, I ran every day for an entire year without missing a day, whether it was raining, sleeting, or snowing, even if I was sick or tired. I thought if I stopped, I'd never be able to start again. I had an "all or nothing" mindset when it came to movement, and it eventually led to shin splints, adrenal fatigue, and eventually burnout. I thought that the only movement that counted was my daily five-mile run. When I was forced to take a break due to a stress fracture, I did nothing for many months. I thought the only meaningful exercise was to run—hard and fast, with my heart pounding, my face red, and sweat pouring off of me. If I couldn't experience that, nothing else mattered. But when my mood tanked and fatigue set in, I realized that if I couldn't run, I had to find other ways keep moving. I couldn't let optimal be the enemy of good enough.

I soon was surprised to learn that every minute I moved my body counted. My body felt good and I lost weight when I shifted from running long distances to practicing yoga, walking, gardening, and doing Pilates.

It's important to remember that with movement, *any* change that improves your life is a good one. If you're doing nothing, doing *something* is the first important step toward living like a PCOS Diva. Find peace in the fact that *something* is always better than *nothing*.

There will be days you'll be able to complete your scheduled hour-long workout. Other days, the only movement you'll get is your 15-minute after-lunch walk, but it's important to remember that the 15-minute walk is better than no walk. At the end of the day, every small step is a victory. It is one more positive choice added to the ever growing set of positive choices you're making.

Finally, please, please don't start down the slippery slope of comparing your movement choices and habits to those of others. Just because your friend is competing in a Tough Mudder doesn't mean that is the right choice for you.

Week Three Weekend Prep: Get a Running Start

Thrive Week is coming! Now is the time to begin planning and prep for Week Three. In addition to your daily food prep this weekend, you'll do your weekend prep. During Weeks One and Two, I provided the meal plans and recipes. Now you are ready branch out and start applying what you have learned.

For Week Three, you will do your own meal planning. Remember that meal planning is an act of self-care. Set aside a bit of time today or tomorrow to craft your meal plan for next week. Use the meal-planning tips in Step 9 of Chapter 6 (p. 108). I've included additional recipes in Chapter 11 (p. 225) for you to use for breakfast, lunch, and dinner as well as more ideas for snacks and sweet treats. Also, there is no shortage of recipe ideas online (including my Seasonal Meal Plans and recipes on PCOSDiva.com) and at your local library or bookstore. Sometimes, I like to grab a cup of tea at my local bookstore, browse through books and magazines for ideas, and work out my Meal Plan while I enjoy a bit of relaxation time.

As you plan, remember to look for recipes that are gluten free, processed-soy free, low-dairy or dairy free, with a good dose of healthy fat, *lots* of veggies, and clean protein. Use the PCOS Diva Plate as a guide.

Sometime during the next day or two, put together your meal plan and shopping list and make time to shop and get yourself prepared for Thrive Week ahead. Also, be sure you look at your calendar for next week and begin scheduling in time for movement as you would doctor's appointments. The more you prep, plan, and schedule, the more successful and lower stress next week will be.

- ☐ Create your own Week Three Meal Plan at a Glance using the meal-planning tips in Step 9 of Chapter 6 (p. 108) to help you.
- ☐ Based upon your Meal Plan, make a detailed list of the grocery items you need for the week, from breakfasts through dinners, including snacks and replacement of staples. Look in your pantry and refrigerator. What do you have on hand and what do you need to put on your shopping list for the next four days?
- ☐ Grocery shop for the next three or four days.
- ☐ Prepare and package snacks for Week Three that can be made in advance.
- ☐ Wash, chop, and store veggies for snacks and salads for the first three or four days.
- ☐ Make a batch or two of homemade salad dressing.
- ☐ Think about your evening food prep. What will you need to do to make it easier to get meals prepared during the week? At the very least, prepare and package snacks and lunch every evening.

Food Prep for Saturday, Day 13

- ☐ Prepare and package snacks.
- ☐ Prepare 10-Layer Salad in a Jar with Citrus Fajitas for lunch.
- ☐ Plan where you will go out to dinner. Review online menus to determine whether the offerings will fit into the Healing PCOS Plan (see Tips for Dining Out, p. 63).

🌿 Day 13

Meal Plan

Breakfast	Snack (Optional)	Lunch	Snack (Required)	Dinner
Apple Pie Smoothie (p. 229)	celery sticks and 2 tablespoons cashew butter with 5 dried cranberries	10-Layer Salad in a Jar (p. 248) with planned-over Citrus Fajitas, guacamole, and salsa	¼ cup 5-Layer Trail Mix (p. 294)	EAT OUT

Inspiration

"Indulgence isn't a sign of failure; it's an opportunity to experience pure pleasure." —Terri Trespicio

Affirmation

"I deserve pleasure."

Diva Daily

Strive to use food as medicine and eat lots of whole foods, because they provide your body with the nutrients and nourishment needed to support health. That said, remember that being a PCOS Diva isn't about deprivation and denial. If you deprive yourself of a food that you really want, chances are that you will eventually binge on the very food you were denying yourself. Deprivation and denial promote disordered eating, and all-or-nothing thinking derails us most often. Think of an indulgence as a food that is not on the daily Healing PCOS Plan, but without ever experiencing it again, life just wouldn't be as sweet. I couldn't imagine life without my grandmother's turkey dressing at the holidays, chocolate-chip ice cream at the beach, or a slice of freshly baked apple pie after an afternoon of apple picking. So, on occasion, give yourself permission to indulge in a few bites of something you really crave, even if it is off the Healing PCOS Plan, without guilt, shame, or remorse.

Diva Do

Eat something "indulgent" with pleasure and without guilt. Here are some guidelines for you to follow.

Know and avoid your "spiral" foods. Spiral foods are the ones you just can't stop eating, and eating them brings no sense of satisfaction. Potato chips are a spiral food for me. One handful is never enough, and I never feel satisfied, even after eating the whole bag. Do not choose a spiral food as an indulgence. In fact, keep spiral foods out of your home.

Don't think of an indulgence as a reward. An indulgence isn't a reward for being "good" all week. An indulgence has a rightful place in the PCOS Diva lifestyle.

Pick a day and plan for an indulgence. As with many things in the PCOS Diva lifestyle, an indulgence should be planned. Planning can take away the guilt and feeling of cheating and allows you to mindfully savor and enjoy the indulgence. In addition, planning gives you something to look forward to, and because you have set the schedule, you are in control. This might mean delaying gratification a bit, which is a good thing. It helps to identify what you really desire. Sunday is typically the day I plan for an indulgence. I'll often make something delicious, usually from the PCOS Diva recipes, for dessert after Sunday dinner.

Be sure your indulgence is worth it. When you really want a chocolate-chip cookie, don't go for the packaged grocery-store version filled with preservatives. Make your own cookies, so you can control the quality of ingredients; try my Chocolate Chip Cookies (p. 300). Enjoy a cookie or two and then share the rest.

Be mindful as you enjoy your indulgence. Take your time, sit down, and avoid distractions. Focus all of your attention on what you are doing and on the food(s) you are eating. Notice the smell, appearance, texture, and taste of the food(s) and the sound as you chew. Relish each bite.

Consider the law of diminishing returns. The law of diminishing returns is an economic principle that says there is a point at which the level of profits or benefits gained decreases with an increase in the amount of money or energy invested. I encourage you to approach your indulgences with this principle in mind. I've found that after three bites of an indulgent dessert, like flourless chocolate cake, the pleasure begins to diminish. This is when I put my fork down. I'm satisfied. I don't feel deprived. I'm in control, and it feels good. I can move forward with no guilt, just contentment.

Record your indulgence. Record the experience in your food journal. Write down how you felt while you were eating the food. Then be sure to check back with yourself two hours after eating. How is your energy compared to before you indulged? How is your mood? Your ability to focus? Do you have any sinus congestion, joint pain, digestive issues, or other physical complaints? You may decide that indulging in certain foods is not worth the trouble. I've learned that often "nothing tastes as good as feeling good feels." That is how I feel about crème brûlée these days. As much as I love it, the bloating and stomach distress I experience after eating it just isn't worth it.

Movement Mindset

Inevitably, there are days when I just don't feel like moving, or I think I'm too busy to dedicate time to movement. Resistance sets in, and I slip back into the all-or-nothing mindset. These resistance busters help to keep me moving:

Give it 10. Getting started is usually the hardest hurdle to clear. But if you can make it through the 5 minutes it takes for you to get ready for a session (changing into appropriate clothing, lacing up your shoes, etc.) and the first 5 minutes of your session, you'll most likely want to keep going. So if you're feeling reluctant to work out, tell yourself you only need to give it 10 minutes—that's nothing!—and then get ready and get started.

Sleep in your workout clothes. If you're in your workout clothes in the morning when the alarm rings, all you have to do is put your feet on the floor, and you are only one move away from getting laced up and off to your workout.

Put money on the line. I schedule my barre workouts for the week ahead using my studio's mobile app. This accountability keeps me on track and gets me to class, because if I cancel less than three hours before class begins, I have to pay the studio $15. In the two years I've gone to barre, I've only paid once. Who wants to lose 15 bucks? Prepay for your training sessions or group fitness workouts or find another way to put money on the line.

Reward yourself. Set up rewards for hitting short-term movement goals. Give yourself something special from your Sweet Stuff list.

Join a group class. My 50-minute barre classes go by in a flash because of the fun music, new exercises, sense of community, and camaraderie. Being in a group of supportive people all working hard together helps me to dig deeper and push a bit harder than I would at home by myself. I feel a connection with the women and instructors at my studio, and it keeps me coming back. Plus, once I am there, I become reenergized.

Find a buddy. Exercise partners provide a powerful combination of support, accountability, motivation, and, in some cases, healthy competition. When you have someone waiting to work out with you, it's a lot harder to make an excuse not to go.

Do something you love. Since I really like Zumba, I don't want to miss class, even though it's early in the morning. It would be much harder to get up so early for a spinning class, since I don't enjoy it.

Use technology. Start a Facebook group with friends, use an app to track your steps, or join an online community to keep you challenged and accountable.

Food Prep for Sunday, Day 14

- ☐ Prepare and package snacks.
- ☐ Think about what you will have for your weekly indulgence. Make plans to bake or cook if needed.
- ☐ Prepare Layered Lunch Wrap with Curried Egg Salad for lunch (put it together in the morning; if it sits overnight it will get soggy).
- ☐ Bake Fruit Scones or wait until morning to prepare.

🌿 Day 14

Meal Plan

Breakfast	Snack (Optional)	Lunch	Snack (Required)	Dinner
Fruit Scone (p. 243)	¼ cup 5-Layer Trail Mix (p. 294)	Layered Lunch Wrap (p. 252) with Curried Egg Salad (p. 252)	½ cup fresh or frozen berries and ¼ cup almonds	Savory Salisbury Steak (p. 262), Root Veggie Mash (p. 279), roasted asparagus (6-Step Roasted Veggies, p. 275), and sliced tomato

Inspiration

"Don't start your day with the broken pieces of yesterday. Every morning we wake up is the first day of the rest of our life." —Anonymous

Affirmation

"I breathe in possibility and breathe out fear."

Diva Daily

Most of the women with PCOS whom I have worked with, myself included, have some level of chronic anxiety. We worry. We take on other people's feelings and energy. Dr. Nancy Dunne helped me reframe this worry and anxiety into "alertness." On my PCOS Diva podcast, she shared, "I'd rather say we are mentally alert, that our nervous systems are in fact turned up a little bit higher. Our sympathetic nervous system is a little bit more reactive when we have a higher androgen status, and in our current culture that can mean things like chronic anxiety and insomnia and eventually depression. It can also be flipped on its other side to give us advantages of perception and motivation to change."

Years ago, I was introduced to the work of Dr. Elaine N. Aron, who has written multiple studies and books on high sensitivity, including *The Highly Sensitive Person*. She also developed a self-test (which you will take in today's Diva Do) to help you determine if you are highly sensitive. She estimates that 15 to 20 percent of people have nervous systems that process stimuli intensely. They think deeply. They feel deeply (physically and emotionally). They easily become overstimulated. Dr. Aron has identified people with higher-tuned nervous systems as highly sensitive persons (HSP) and asserts that they are genetically predisposed to be more aware and empathic. Dr. Aron has studied this phenomenon extensively and, using MRI brain scans, she's found that highly sensitive people experience sounds, feelings, and even the presence of other people much more intensely than the average person.

I've tried to describe to my husband the way I feel when I am overstimulated by noise, emotion, too many things on my to-do list, and other people's negative energy. The only way that seems to make sense to him is to think of me as a computer that is processing so much information that it starts acting glitchy and freezes. Like that computer, I need to reboot by taking a nap, going to acupuncture, taking a bath, or a walk in nature or doing another form of self-care. Once I've shut down for a little while, I'm restored and can operate more efficiently.

I no longer see being mentally alert or highly sensitive as a limitation. It is an asset as long as I know how to support myself. Being highly sensitive is a characteristic of a truly alive and compassionate human being.

Diva Do

Take Dr. Aron's Highly Sensitive Person Test (hsperson.com). If you score 14 points or more, you are part of the club.

Knowing that I am a highly sensitive person was a huge "aha" moment on my journey. *Self-awareness is an important part of living like a PCOS Diva, because it helps you assess what you really need to practice better self-care.* If you are a highly sensitive person, many of the Diva Daily lessons will help you manage your more alert and sensitive nervous system. Successful highly sensitive PCOS Divas practice habits that truly nourish them.

Movement Mindset

Planning is key in all areas of the PCOS Diva lifestyle. Planning your meals, shopping lists, and movement creates momentum and sustainability and sets you up for success. During Week Three, you will plan your own movement. So let's do some homework now to make that process easier for you. Today you will work on your Movement Menu.

Come up with a list of various ways you can move your body for different time intervals. Describe your choices just like a menu in a fine restaurant:

Appetizer: A movement that takes 5 minutes or less

Entree: Longer sustained movement

Dessert: A short and really pleasurable movement

Most people don't realize that it is not the "work" part of exercise they hate; it's how boring the activity is. If this sounds like you, try to remember how you liked to move as a girl. Did you dance, do gymnastics, play basketball? Recalling those activities will get you back in touch with how your body likes to move. Keep this in mind as you create your Movement Menu. In addition, include activities you would like to try, such as a Zumba class or hot yoga.

Here are some samples from which to choose to create your Movement Menu:

Appetizers

- Dancing to favorite song
- Planking for 90 seconds
- 15 pushups
- 30 squats
- 10 burpees

Entrees

- 35-minute power walk
- HIIT circuit
- 60-minute hike
- 50-minute exercise class
- 40-minute bike ride
- 30-minute Zumba routine
- 25 minutes on a rebounder while catching up on favorite show

Dessert

- 10-minute restorative yoga routine
- Walking around the block
- Using a foam roller
- 10-minute stretch
- Playing tag with kids for 10 minutes
- Walking the dog

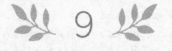

9

Week Three:

THRIVE

You are unique and beautiful, and you deserve to heal and *thrive*. You're moving, eating, and, most important, thinking like a PCOS Diva. Now you are going to thrive like a PCOS Diva, continuously flourishing and transcending the pain and struggle of PCOS to live the life you are meant to live and share your unique gifts with the world.

You've come so far in the past two weeks. You've made great choices, and you're feeling better as a result. Take a moment to reflect upon and celebrate the new habits you've incorporated into your daily routine, such as drinking lemon water and dry brushing, and how, collectively, these small habits are adding up to a healthy new lifestyle and a healthier version of yourself. Celebrate the times you chose to drink a smoothie rather than eat a break-room donut, ordered a PCOS Diva–friendly meal rather than an unhealthy choice at a restaurant, or took a walk after lunch instead of staying in and scrolling through Facebook. Celebrate the return of your energy and the improvement in the way you feel.

During Week Three, you will build upon the lessons learned in the past two weeks. You will follow the same daily protocol and add a key new component of self-care: meditation. You will wake up 5 to

10 minutes earlier this week to create space in your daily routine to add a Meditation Moment in the morning. I like to say that I start my day with M and M's: movement and meditation.

I used to think meditation was just for yogis and hippies, but I have found that it is a really easy way to become more mindful, more centered, and less anxious; most important, it helps me manage stress. *Stress is at the root of most doctor visits and is a trigger for the three most common symptoms of PCOS: insulin resistance and hyperinsulinemia, hormonal imbalance, and chronic inflammation.* Research shows that prolonged stress releases the hormone cortisol, which reduces cell function and contributes to numerous emotional and physical disorders. Most alarming for women with PCOS, cortisol increases sugar (glucose) in the bloodstream, while suppressing immune system responses, the digestive system, and the reproductive system.

Meditation isn't only for stress relief, though. Studies indicate that people who engage in mind–body interventions of any kind (yoga, tai chi, etc.) see benefits on the genetic level. This type of activity seems to cause a reduction of activity in genes associated with inflammation. The National Institutes of Health agrees that meditation can be useful for reducing high blood pressure and symptoms of irritable bowel syndrome and ulcerative colitis. It may also ease symptoms of anxiety, depression, and pain while enhancing mood and self-esteem and even helping with insomnia. For all of these reasons and more, we will make meditation a part of our day.

It can be used just about anytime or anywhere to recenter yourself and work through overwhelming moments. You don't have to be in a silent room with a yogi. You can meditate at your desk, on a train, in the shower, on a walk, or in a room full of screaming children. Just take a minute or two and focus on your breathing.

There are many types of meditation, and no one method is ideal for everyone. The best meditation is the one that works for you. You'll learn about seven different types of meditation this week in our Meditation Moments, with the goal of discovering the types you enjoy and work best for you. Maybe you can't imagine sitting on a meditation pillow with fingers posed, chanting "Om." That is okay, because there are lots of other ways to meditate and reap the benefits.

Although "Thrive" week is the final week of the 21-Day Plan, it is not the end of your journey. Thriving like a PCOS Diva is a road of perpetual growth. The road isn't always straight, it may not be smooth traveling, and there will be twists and turns, but you will reap the benefits of the growth you experience along the way. From now on, you will strive each day to grow into a healthier, happier, and fuller version of yourself.

You know the old saying, "Give a man a fish and you feed him for a day. Teach a man to fish and you feed him for a lifetime." This week you are going to learn to fish, so to speak. You will choose recipes and create your own Meal Plan. Please don't underestimate the power of planning. Create your Meal Plan and shopping list, and go grocery shopping. Also, be sure to plan out your movement and self-care for the week. Put it on your calendar and treat it as you would a doctor's appointment. It is that important!

You can do this. You know enough. You are enough. Keep putting one foot in front of the other and taking steps forward.

Thrive: Week Three Daily Protocol

☐ Bonus Movement: HIIT added to walk(s), 10 minutes of strength training, or 10 minutes of mind–body exercise sometime during the day

Rocket Launch. *Wake up 5–10 minutes earlier than last week.*
    ☐ Morning Motto
    ☐ Big Why
    ☐ Gratitude

Morning Reflection
    ☐ Morning elixir
    ☐ Inspiration
    ☐ Affirmation
    ☐ 15-minute Morning Movement
    ☐ Meditation Moment

Shower
    ☐ Dry brushing before shower
    ☐ Oil massage after shower

Breakfast
- ☐ Meal
- ☐ Breakfast supplements
- ☐ Tongue scrape

Daily Lesson
- ☐ Diva Daily
- ☐ Diva Do

Morning Snack/Tea Time
- ☐ Optional snack
- ☐ Beverage break

Lunch
- ☐ Meal
- ☐ Lunch supplements
- ☐ 15-minute walk

Afternoon Snack/Tea Time
- ☐ Required snack
- ☐ Beverage break
- ☐ Water check (have you had enough water today?)

Dinner
- ☐ Meal
- ☐ Dinner supplements
- ☐ 15-minute walk
- ☐ Dessert chocolate (optional)
- ☐ Next day food prep

Nighttime Ritual
- ☐ Unplugged by 8 p.m.
- ☐ Evening elixir and/or evening snack (only if needed)
- ☐ Tomorrow's Priority List
- ☐ Magnesium
- ☐ Tongue scrape
- ☐ Essential oils
- ☐ Stretching
- ☐ Book
- ☐ Gratitude stone
- ☐ Sleep mask and lights out by 10 p.m.

🌿 Day 15

Inspiration

"You teach the people around you how to treat you. They learn by watching how you treat yourself." —Kimberley Jones

Affirmation

"I attract positive energy like a magnet."

Meditation Moment

You have been working to create a *movement* mindset, but you will also be developing a *meditation* mindset. Look for opportunities that you might otherwise spend dwelling on the negative or creating anxiety and worry, and use them for a mindful Meditation Moment.

Meditation practices are invaluable for dealing with stress. You've learned how stress wreaks havoc on PCOS. We can't always eliminate stressors from our lives, but we *can* learn to manage the stress in healthier ways. *Breathing Breaks* are a great tool. We take twenty-five thousand breaths every day, but I would bet that many of us rarely take more than a couple deep breaths during an entire day, even when we're *not* feeling stressed.

Breathing is an automatic function controlled by the autonomic nervous system. This nervous system consists of two parts: the sympathetic and the parasympathetic systems. The sympathetic is the "fight or flight" system. It prepares the body for sudden stress by controlling physical things like our heart rate, adrenal glands, and breathing. The parasympathetic system prepares the body to "rest and digest" and activates the more tranquil functions of the body, helping the digestive system work more efficiently to extract nutrients from our food.

When we are stressed out, overworked, or overstimulated during our daily lives, we are in a chronic state of fight or flight. Our breathing becomes short, sharp, shallow, and quick; we may barely breathe at all. In turn our minds become anxious, nervous, and agitated. But we can work to consciously shift the body into the parasympathetic rest-and-digest mode just by using our breath. It's a simple technique, and it's so powerful. Slow, deep breathing can instantly calm us down mentally as well as physically.

Set your phone alarm for three separate 1-minute Breathing Breaks today.

Breathing Break

1. Set the timer for 1 minute so you can focus on breathing and let the time take care of itself.
2. Place your left hand on your upper chest and your right hand on your belly, in the space just below your rib cage.
3. Inhale through your nose slowly and strongly right down into your belly, pushing your right hand softly outward. If your left hand is moving, your breathing is too shallow; it is in your chest, and you are not breathing into your belly as you should. Let the air completely fill your lungs. Just when you think you cannot inhale any more, try to sip in one last bit.
4. Hold the breath for a moment.
5. Begin to exhale through your nose, pushing the air out of your stomach and pulling your belly in toward your spine. Exhale all of the breath in your lungs.
6. Take another full deep breath in through your nose, hold, and exhale completely. Try to exhale for twice as long as you inhale, and fully expel the air. When you breathe in and out, your left hand should remain still and only your right hand should move up and down.
7. Continue breathing in this way until 1 minute is up.

I love using these tools to help with my Breathing Breaks:

- *Spire.* The Spire is a breath and activity tracker. It is a little smooth, stonelike clip that you attach to your bra or waistband. The Spire identifies periods when your breathing reflects a tense state of mind and vibrates when it detects several minutes of tense breathing. The device sends a message to an app on your smartphone to remind you to breathe. It interrupts the cycle of tension and anxiety and reminds you to take a Breathing Break. This device has helped me to become aware of my own breath, and as a result I'm less anxious, calmer, and more centered throughout the day.

- *Inner Balance monitor.* Heartmath's Inner Balance sensor measures heart rhythms rather than breath using a little probe that you clip on your earlobe and connect to a smartphone app. You can then use the app to sync your breathing with your heart rate.

- *There's an app for that.* Although not specifically focused on just breathing, countless apps are available to guide you through many types of meditation. For many, this simplifies meditation, since it takes the responsibility for timing and planning away from meditators and allows them to give themselves completely to the experience. My favorites are TheMindfulnessApp.com, Headspace.com, and Calm.com.

Throughout the week, you will take Meditation Moments that focus on breathing. Please try the techniques I mentioned above. Not only do Breathing Breaks help combat stress, but they also create mindfulness. Focusing on your breath places you in the "now." We cannot breathe in the past, and we cannot yet breathe in the future. We must breathe in the now moment. Paying attention to your breath allows your mind to become more present-moment focused.

Diva Daily

Surround yourself with people who want you to thrive. *You deserve to spend your time with people who lift you up.* Invest in relationships that energize you. Spend time with people who are focused on becoming the best version of themselves, who move forward with gratitude while growing, getting better, and maximizing their potential. They say you are the sum of the five people you spend the most time with. Make sure they're positive!

Steer clear of negative people. These are the folks who relish the negative things in their life and the lives of others and ignore the positive.

They exaggerate issues they are facing, making their predicament seem a lot worse than it is. Negative people are exhausting to be around. Their energy depletes rather than invigorates. You cannot thrive if you are surrounded by negative people.

Diva Do

Take out your journal and write down all of the people in your life you interact with on a daily, weekly, and monthly basis. Next to their names, write what type of "S" they are. Do they Suck from you? Do you feel energetically depleted when you spend time with them? Do they Sabotage you and try to keep you from living life like a PCOS Diva by tempting you with gluten-laden sweets? Or do they Support you? Do they Stretch you to meet your goals and thrive, to become the best version of yourself? The latter are the people you need to spend more time with!

Then begin to create boundaries around those who Suck and Sabotage. If you are a highly sensitive person, you will keenly feel the negative effects of people who Suck and Sabotage and you'll need to take extra precautions to protect yourself. You will have to set some boundaries and practice saying no when you don't want to do something with them because you know that you will end up exhausted, depleted, or overwhelmed. Be mindful of flexing your "no" muscle this week with those who keep you from thriving.

Day 16

Inspiration

"Balance isn't something you find. It's something you create."
—Jana Kingsford

Affirmation

"I enjoy a well-balanced lifestyle."

Meditation Moment

I use the 5 to 10 minutes I spend in the shower as an opportunity to cleanse my body as well as my mind and spirit. I let the water wash away my fears, worries, and problems, right down the drain. As with body brushing, mindfulness and meditation in the shower are great ways to become more comfortable with our bodies, in the present moment, without judgment. Enjoy what a simple mindful pleasure a shower can be.

The time you spend in the shower is the perfect opportunity for a Meditation Moment. You are alone and away from the distractions of life, if only for a few minutes, and a few minutes are all that you need for a *Shower Meditation*.

Shower Meditation

1. Prepare your towel, after-bath oils, and any other items you need after your shower.
2. Set your intention that you are not just cleaning your body, but your mind and spirit as well.
3. Feel the water as it hits your skin. Take a moment to be thankful for the warm running water.
4. As water is falling on you, close your eyes and focus on your breath. Inhale and feel the cleansing warm steam flow in through your nose. Exhale and release your negative thoughts, stress, tensions, and feelings of being overwhelmed. Imagine these thoughts dissolving in the water and floating down the drain. Take six more deep breaths like this.
5. Proceed with your shower. As you wash, smell the aroma of the soap and listen to the water flow. Acutely feel the soap against your skin, feel your fingers rubbing the shampoo into your scalp. As you scrub each body part, give thanks for what it brings to you and enables you to do.
6. When you're finished washing, take a few deeper breaths, focusing on the sensation of the water before you turn it off. You should feel more centered, calm, rejuvenated, and ready to take on your day.

Diva Daily

In order to thrive, we must become more self-aware and make time for self-reflection. An important question to ask is "Where do I need more balance in my life?" What areas of your life need more attention, so you can flourish? As a coach, I love using my Thrive like a PCOS Diva Wheel to help clients determine where they need to create more balance in their life. It is not meant to be a report card on how well you have performed or what you have achieved. It is meant to take a snapshot of a specific moment. The wheel reveals how balanced your life is right now.

The Thrive like a PCOS Diva Wheel (p. 202) is divided into ten sections, each of which has a scale that goes from 0 in the center to 10 at the outer edge. Lower numbers mean little balance in an area, while higher ones indicate the presence of more balance. Place a dot on the scale representing your rating for each area. When you've rated all areas on the wheel, connect the dots to form an inner wheel, a visual representation of the balance in your life right now. It is unlikely that all areas in your life are perfect 10s; everyone will have a wheel that is lopsided to some degree. However, you'll find that the rounder and more balanced your wheel is, the easier the ride and the more you thrive and are able move forward in your life. If your wheel was on a bike, how bumpy would your ride be?

Diva Do

Take a few minutes to fill out your Thrive like a PCOS Diva Wheel. Connect the dots and see how it looks. Which segments have the lowest scores? Where do you need more balance in your life? Remember, the goal isn't to have all perfect 10s. The goal is for your circle to resemble a wheel. Focus on the lowest scoring segment. What action can you take today to help you go up a notch? Write down the item and commit to taking action before the end of the day. Make it a point to do this exercise once a month. It is satisfying to see your progress.

Day 17

Inspiration

"Most of the shadows of this life are caused by standing in one's own sunshine." —Ralph Waldo Emerson

Affirmation

"I love myself as I am."

Meditation Moment

Walking Meditation is one of my favorite ways to center myself and alleviate stress and anxiety. The repetition of the movement helps me to stay in the present and quiet my mind. My mind follows the rhythm of walking instead of getting lost in my thoughts. This kind of walk will change your day for the better.

Walking Meditation

1. Map out a route. A nature trail is best.
2. Don't listen to music, and turn your cell phone on vibrate. You want to hear the sound of your breath and the subtle sounds of the natural world around you.
3. Begin to move in concert with your breath. Become aware of your breath. Try to inhale for three steps and exhale for three steps. Make sure that the length of the inhale matches the length of the exhale.
4. Sense your movement. Focus on the experience of walking, the sensations in your feet and legs, your arms swinging, your whole body moving. Pay attention to each foot as it makes contact with the ground. Hear the rhythm of your feet hitting the ground.
5. Try not to look around, but rather gaze out in front of you.
6. To take this meditation a step farther, focus on your blessings and think about all the things you are grateful for, for example, your relationships, your body, and abilities like the simple act of being able to walk.

Thrive like a PCOS Diva Wheel

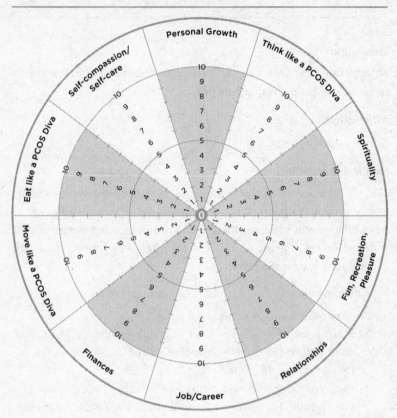

Spirituality

- I am connected with something bigger than myself.
- I take time for a spiritual practice.
- I forgive others and myself.
- I take time to feed my spirit through meditation, introspection, reading, and reflection.
- I practice gratitude.
- I spend time in nature.

Think like a PCOS Diva

- I practice progress rather than perfection.
- I take control rather than act like a victim.
- I partner with and listen to my body.
- I think from a place of abundance rather than from a place of lack.
- I am authentic.
- I am enough.

Self-compassion/Self-care

- My internal dialogue is more positive than negative.
- I treat myself to Sweet Stuff.
- I take extreme self-care.
- I appreciate myself.
- I am kind to myself.
- I schedule time for myself.

Personal Growth

- I know my unique strengths and gifts.
- I use my creativity.
- I share my gifts with others.
- I am continually learning new things.
- I enjoy new opportunities for growth.
- I am growing and flourishing as a person.

Eat like a PCOS Diva

- I sizzle in the kitchen.
- I am a PCOS Diva when eating out.
- I plan meals and create a shopping list.
- I use food as medicine.
- I take my supplements.
- I eat fresh seasonal produce.

Move like a PCOS Diva

- I move my body in ways that feel good.
- I am not exhausted every time I practice my preferred movement.
- I move my body every day.
- I combine HIIT, strength training, and mind–body exercise each week.
- I get adequate sleep.
- I move because I love my body, not to punish myself.

Finances

- I earn enough money.
- I live beneath my means.
- I have money and resources to pursue my goals.
- I save for the future.
- I plan for financial freedom.
- I am grateful for all I have.

Job/Career

- I am happy at my job.
- My job aligns with the PCOS Diva lifestyle.
- I have room to grow.
- My job aligns with my gifts and strengths.
- My job is personally and financially satisfying.
- My work nourishes me.

Relationships

- I spend time with those who support and stretch me.
- I set boundaries with negative people who suck my energy and sabotage my success.
- I nurture relationships with positive and supportive people.
- I am happy with my social circle.
- I am my authentic self.
- I say no when I need to.

Fun, Recreation, Pleasure

- I have fun often.
- I enjoy sports or other hobbies.
- I indulge mindfully when eating.
- I make time for rest and renewal.
- I find ways to express my creativity.
- I give myself permission to experience pleasure.

Diva Daily

When I was really struggling with PCOS, I had lost all sense of how my appearance and the clothes I wore could reflect my true self. I had spent eight years in the corporate world, wearing business attire on most days. When my first child was born, I became a stay-at-home mom. I went from an aspiring business executive to a "frumpy mom" who mostly wore sweats and her husband's old T-shirts. As a frumpy mom, I didn't think I was worth spending money and time on to dress beautifully. This went on for several years. It's no coincidence that my health took a dive. The less I cared about my appearance, the less I cared about what I ate or other aspects of self-care. I was caught in a place of lack—not enough, time, money, or energy to take care of myself—and my health spiraled downward.

One of the things that helped stop the downward spiral was to begin putting effort into my appearance again. When I did, I stopped wallowing and started moving forward and upward. I was less likely to eat poorly, avoid having my picture taken, hide from mirrors, and withdraw from social invitations. I began to thrive.

Rediscovering and expressing my personal style through fashion helped me rediscover my confidence and power. I began showing up in the world differently, self-assured and strong. I became more present in my body, treating it with more care. I stopped comparing myself to others. I worked to highlight my best features and found what worked best for me and my body type. I realized that when I was overly critical of my body, it undermined my ability to feel beautiful. By changing the way I dressed, I changed the relationship I had with my body for the better. More self-love begets more self-care, and self-care is elemental to thriving.

Diva Do

Are you dressing like the PCOS Diva you are? If not, then let's get to work on discovering your personal style. Personal style is an extension of who you are. It is your personal brand that communicates who you are without saying a word. How do you want to project yourself? Looking perfect isn't the end goal; it is about feeling good. Clothes can make us feel beautiful. Find what makes *you* feel beautiful.

Look for inspiration. Make your own "look book." I think the easiest way to do this is to create a Pinterest board. Trust your gut and pin images you feel attracted to and styles that you love. Don't edit yourself. Just keep pinning. The more you just follow your gut, the faster this will go. After a while, you'll start to see trends emerge. Look at the color palette you are attracted to. What kind of textures do you like? Do a board for each season. After you've "brainstormed" your style board, edit it, and take out anything you don't really love. Use your "look book" as a reference when you go shopping.

Clear out what no longer serves. We all have that one pair of jeans in our closet that we hold on to, hoping we can squeeze into them again one day. Let's embrace who we are in this moment. Get rid of those "maybe one day" items in your closet. Remove anything that doesn't fit. Give the items away, and if you just can't part with them, put them in storage somewhere else. Next, clear out anything that you don't like, haven't worn in over a year, and aren't excited to put on. Finally, ask, "Does this fit my emerging personal style? Does it align with the PCOS Diva I'm becoming?" If the answer is yes, then keep it.

Ask a professional. Leave it to the experts; they know what they are doing. I've come to rely on my favorite boutiques and free professional stylist services offered at many department stores to help me find clothes that fit my personal style. Personal style doesn't have to be expensive. Shop the sale racks. I typically show the stylist my latest "look book," and she helps select clothes in my price range that make me feel great. I've also discovered that online services such as Stitch Fix can take the time and frustration out of shopping, identify clothes that I love, and help develop my personal style.

What I really want for you is to *feel* as beautiful as you *are.* Ultimately, everything in your closet should:

- Fit well. Do not fall into the squeeze-into-the-smallest-size mindset. You are beautiful in whatever size fits.
- Be worn often.
- Be comfortable and feel good.
- Represent the image you want to project to the world.

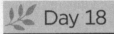 Day 18

Inspiration

"What you hold on to holds on to you. Is it loving, kind, and empowering? Does it make you feel good about yourself? If not, let it go."
—Anna Pereira

Affirmation

"My life is filled with beauty and organization."

Meditation Moment

I love fresh flowers. Every week as part of my Sweet Stuff indulgences, I treat myself to fresh-cut flowers that I arrange and keep in a vase on my kitchen island. They lift my spirits, and gazing upon them can help calm my frazzled nerves and center me in anticipation of a busy day ahead. *Flower Gazing* is the simplest Meditation Moment imaginable.

Flower Gazing

1. Choose a flower, with a single blossom, that inspires you.
2. Sit in a chair where you can gaze upon the flower about 16 inches in front of you. You can hold the flower or place it in a bud vase.
3. Relax your facial muscles. Gaze upon the flower with soft, relaxed eyes, without allowing your eyes to break contact.
4. While gazing, take a Breathing Break and take slow deep breaths.
5. Stare for 15 to 20 seconds at a minimum. Work your way up to 5 minutes or more.
6. If your attention wanders from focusing on the flower, simply notice that it happened, then bring yourself back to gazing. When thoughts pop into your head, acknowledge them, then gently redirect your attention back to the flower in front of you.
7. Before you are finished, generate feelings of gratitude for the gifts of healing and beauty of the flower and offer thanks for its beauty and replenishment.

8. Finally, close your eyes for a minute or so. Can you still see its image in your mind or feel its presence in front of you?
9. During this meditation, don't be surprised if you begin to yawn, even if you are not tired, or tears form in your eyes. Both are signs of stress release.

Diva Daily

Clearing out the clutter in our life helps us get a clearer idea of who we are and what we truly want. Physical clutter, anything not needed anymore or disorganized, distracts and paralyzes us from moving forward to our next chapter in life. Mess causes stress. It drags our energy down, and we experience feelings of anxiety, being overwhelmed, exhaustion, and even depression. Research shows that clutter may even cause us to overeat!

Clutter slowly creeps up. It begins with a pile here and a junk drawer there until it becomes a distraction, a literal barrier. A study on organized and cluttered living by the Princeton University Neuroscience Institute concluded that if you want to focus to the best of your abilities, you need to clear clutter from your home and work environment. Decluttering and organizing your home can help you to be less irritable, more productive, and less distracted. Clutter caused people to lose focus and brain-processing power.

Decluttering helps us thrive, emotionally, spiritually, and mentally. It reduces stress, simplifies our life, releases energy that has been buried under things belonging to our past, and allows for new possibilities. We would clean up our home if we had company coming to stay. Why not treat ourselves like those special guests? Decluttering is an act of self-care. You deserve it. You are worth having beautiful, clean, and uncluttered spaces.

Diva Do

Focus on something in your home to declutter. If you haven't tackled your kitchen yet, begin with a kitchen drawer or cabinet. Estimate how much time it might take to complete the task and set a timer. Having a finite amount of time for the task will help you stay focused. If you aren't sure, start with 15 minutes. Notice how you feel looking at the disorganized, cluttered drawer. Does it make you feel anxious? Does your energy feel stagnant?

It's time to eliminate what is old or unnecessary or doesn't reflect who you are any longer. Take everything out of the drawer and create three piles:

1. Things to throw away.
2. Things to give away.
3. Things to keep. Only keep what you really need or want.

If you have a hard time throwing or giving things away, challenge yourself to find at least three things to eliminate from that space. Clean the drawer or cabinet, making sure it is free from stains or dust and place your kept items back in an organized way.

After finishing the short decluttering project, take a moment and check in with yourself. How do you feel? Do you feel lighter, freer? Calmer? Do you feel more energetic? If you've got some momentum from doing that one space, then keep going. Tackle something else, but complete one area at a time. Consider taking on a drawer, closet, or area of your home every day for the next 21 days.

Day 19

Inspiration

"The things you are passionate about are not random. They are your calling." —Fabienne Fredrickson

Affirmation

"Being creative makes me feel alive."

Meditation Moment

Coloring can be a form of meditation that taps into your creativity at the same time. Dr. Joel Pearson, a brain scientist at the University of New South Wales in Australia, believes that concentrating on coloring an image may facilitate the replacement of negative thoughts and images with pleasant ones. A 2005 study concurred, demonstrating that coloring mandalas may induce a meditative state that benefits individuals suffering from anxiety. *Coloring Meditation* helps me tune out the chaos of the day as I focus on a single, soothing, and creative activity.

Give yourself 15 minutes. Print out a coloring sheet (there are tons online), grab some colored pencils, put on some relaxing music, and color away.

Diva Daily

Through my personal experience and coaching many women with PCOS, I have discovered a surprising common denominator in women who are struggling with their symptoms. They have lost touch with their ability to creatively express themselves. When I look back on my life, I have come to realize that during the periods when I was thriving, I was creating. When I began feeling better in college, I was not only cooking, eating, and exercising more effectively; I was also reconnected with my creativity. I was an art-history major and had to take two semesters of studio-arts classes. I am no artist, but getting lost in the studio, creating with paints and canvas was soothing to my soul. It was a way to practice mindfulness and a great stress reducer. When I'm nurturing my creative spirit, I thrive.

When we lose touch with our creative power, our PCOS symptoms may increase. Studies have shown that art therapy and creative engagement can decrease anxiety, stress, and mood disturbances. Start reconnecting with your creative power, and you will begin to thrive, I promise.

Diva Do

Remember making art as a child? Like me, you probably lost yourself in the moment as you finger-painted, played with Play-Doh, or colored. You were in a state of "flow." Your senses were heightened, and you were in the moment, with no concept of time. In a flow state, there is a dimming of the external world, and we are excited about what we are experiencing. We are fully alive. I call that thriving.

But sadly, as we grow up, we often stop making art and lose that flow state. We lose touch with our creativity. It is time to reclaim your creative power. You can tap into it through a variety of ways: dance, drama, music, writing, crafting, scrapbooking, coloring, quilting, photography, cooking, and more. What form of art calls to you? Think back to when you were last lost in a state of flow. What were you doing?

Commit to expressing your creativity in some way by the end of this week. Give yourself a solid block of creating time and consider adding creative pursuits to your Sweet Stuff list. Experiment with artistic pursuits without judging yourself too critically. Treat yourself as you would a child. You would never criticize a young child's creative work. Perfectionism is the killer of creativity. Notice if you begin judging your creative project from a place of "This isn't good enough," or "I'm not doing it right." Also, creativity isn't a linear process. You don't have to have an end goal. Rather, start just for pleasure. Enjoy the process, experience, and create. You deserve to have fun and heal.

🌿 Day 20

Inspiration

"A moment of self-compassion can change your entire day. A string of such moments can change the course of your life."
—Christopher K. Germer

Affirmation

"I treat myself with kindness."

Meditation Moment

One of my favorite ways to pause and meditate is based upon a *metta* meditation, or *Loving-Kindness Meditation*. *Metta* is Pali, the language of the Buddhist canon, for "friendliness" or "kindness." This type of meditation has been shown to increase positive emotions and decrease negative ones and helps reduce self-criticism. Give yourself 5 minutes of kindness. If you practice this meditation often, I promise you will feel more self-compassion.

Loving-Kindness Meditation

1. Get comfortable in a chair with feet grounded on the floor. I like to put my hands in prayer pose over my heart. Close your eyes and start by taking 4 Box Breaths. Inhale in for 4 counts, hold for 4 counts, exhale for 4 counts, rest for 4 counts, and then repeat for a total of 4 breaths. Focus on feeling love and kindness for yourself. Imagine your heart center radiating a warm, glowing light. Let any negative feelings of self-judgment and self-hatred go from your awareness.

2. While continuing to take deep breaths, think of and ask for the good and loving things that you want more of in your life, while working on connecting with those good feelings. Extend grace and kindness to yourself. Say:

   May I be happy.

   May I be healthy.

   May I be safe.

   May I be blessed.

3. Direct your attention to the part of yourself that feels out of sorts or disconnected, and say to yourself four times, "May that part be of me be filled with kindness," and then say four times, "May my whole body be filled with kindness."

4. Then do one more round of Box Breathing and say, "May I be happy, may I be healthy, may I be safe, may I be blessed." Slowly open your eyes and come out of the meditation.

Diva Daily

How can we thrive if we are not being kind to ourselves? If self-love seems too lofty right now, then start with self-compassion.

Think about the last time you made a mistake or messed up, even if it was something small. What did you say to yourself? "I'll never succeed," "I always mess things up," "I'm a failure," or "I'll never be enough"? Would you ever speak that way to someone you truly care about? If you kept track of all the self-berating thoughts you have each day, you might be shocked. When these thoughts are woven into our internal fabric day after day, our reality begins to take shape based upon those thoughts. You are so much more than those old negative thinking patterns would allow you to believe. Stop being so hard on yourself. Think about this: the longest relationship you will ever have is with yourself; make it a positive one.

You are allowed to make mistakes. Work hard to treat yourself kindly and show as much empathy, mercy, and tenderness toward yourself as you would toward your child or dear friend. Embrace your imperfections, and dare to be vulnerable. Instead of punishing yourself, consider missteps a learning experience or an opportunity to grow. Learn the lessons, so you can move forward in life. Don't take yourself and every situation too seriously. Sometimes you might just need to brush off a mistake and find a way to laugh about it. You'll be amazed where a little self-compassion can take you.

Diva Do

Take 10 minutes today to sit down and write yourself a letter of encouragement. Think about all you have accomplished over the last twenty days. Be your own cheerleader and revel in your successes. Savoring life's joys and victories will make the good last longer and the negative seem less important. If you find those perfectionist tendencies surfacing or the negative ticker tape rolling, and you are feeling as though you are not enough, then use this as an opportunity for some self-compassion.

Think of a time during the last three weeks when you felt "not enough." Describe how the incident made you feel. Did you feel shame, anger, guilt, embarrassment? Keep this incident in mind, and add to your encouragement letter a bit of compassion, understanding, and acceptance for the part of yourself that you felt was lacking. Avoid judging yourself, and write as if you are giving advice to a dear friend you love unconditionally. Ask yourself what you could do in the future to improve this negative aspect. Focus on how a small shift or positive step forward could help you thrive, feel happier and healthier, and avoid judging yourself.

Read this letter from time to time (especially in challenging times) as a reminder to be more self-compassionate.

Day 21

Inspiration

"We often wish and pray for mountains of difficulty to be removed, when we should be praying for the courage to climb them." —Anonymous

Affirmation

"I am courageous."

Meditation Moment

The Emotional Freedom Technique (EFT), otherwise known as *Tapping,* is a tool that has vastly improved my stress levels and quality of life, helped me move beyond fear, and eased my anxiety and worry. EFT was developed by Stanford engineer Gary Craig in 1993. EFT is a specific algorithm for "tapping" on energy meridian end points, which sends a calming response to the body.

You may be wondering how tapping on "energy meridians" can help with anxiety and overall well-being. If you think about it, our bodies haven't changed all that much from those of our hunter-gatherer ancestors. When we feel threatened or endangered, the part of the brain called the amygdala begins to fire off, and we go into fight-or-flight mode. This is the area of the brain where the stress response begins. On a moment's notice, our body reacts to a perceived threat by increasing our heart rate and pumping adrenaline through our body. Our muscles tense up, and our body is ready to either fight or run away.

The problem we face in this modern day is that our amygdala cannot tell the difference between a real threat or a perceived one, so getting into a heated discussion with your boss can create the same physical response our ancestors had when faced with a wild beast. Tapping on the end points of meridians sends a calming response to the body, and the amygdala recognizes that it's safe. Science supports this too. Research at Harvard Medical School over the past decade has shown that stimulation of selected meridian acupressure points decreases activity in the amygdala.

To take it one step farther, doing the tapping while imagining or discussing a stressful event counteracts that stress and reprograms the response to it. When you focus on your stressor while you tap on the energy meridian end points or acupressure points, you will find that you can have the same thought but without having the physical anxiety. This allows you to easily let go of whatever stressor or negative thought is bothering you by replacing it with a much more empowering thought.

Tapping may seem strange at first and may take a bit of practice. The first thing is learning the meridian end points, or tapping points.

Karate-chop point, located below your pinky on the soft part of the outside of your hand

Eyebrow point, located in the inside corner of your eye socket right where the hair of your eyebrow begins.

Side of the eye, located on the outside corner of the eye socket at the side of the eye (it's not on the temple; it's actually on the bone).

Under the eye, located on the bone just underneath your eye.

Under the nose, located under your nose, between your nose and lip.

Chin, not the chin point, but located on the crease between your lip and your chin.

Collar bone, located in the center of the upper part of your chest where a man's bowtie would lie (tap here with your entire hand).

Under the arm, located under your arm, located about 4 inches below your armpit

Top of the head.

Tapping

1. *Rate your issue.* Give your feeling, whether it's physical or emotional, a rating on a scale of 1 to 10. If you're tapping on a physical symptom, ask yourself, "On a scale of 1 to 10, how painful is it, 10 being very painful and 1 I barely feel it." When measuring emotions, you can ask yourself, "How much anxiety do I feel on a scale of 1 to 10?"

2. *Craft a setup statement.* Create a statement that expresses your stressor and then your unconditional acceptance of or love for yourself. Here is an example: "Even though I am anxious about the presentation I am giving tomorrow, I accept myself." There are different variations to the second part. Some people say, "I love and accept myself," or "I accept myself and how I feel." It's not really about using the perfect words. It's about saying the words that bring up the emotion and energy (fear, anxiety, worry, or physical pain) that you want to clear. I hope through this program you've become more comfortable with talking to yourself from a place of love, but it may still seem foreign to you. Perhaps you fear that accepting yourself means you accept your current situation, so nothing will change, yet it's often our inability to accept ourselves that keeps us stuck.

3. *Tap on tapping points.* While you tap with your four fingers on the karate-chop point for five to seven times, repeat the setup statement three times. Then begin to tap on other points, beginning with the top of your head. Tap with your fingers on one side or the other or both together (I prefer both) five to seven times at each point while simply saying how you feel. Be honest with how you feel. Take a deep breath once you have finished the sequence.

4. *Rate your issue.* Rate the intensity of your issue again. Repeat until you get the relief you desire.

Diva Daily

Chances are when you got your PCOS diagnosis, fear was your first emotion. I know it was mine. Knowing that I had an incurable chronic health condition that could ultimately lead to cardiovascular disease, type 2 diabetes, and fertility struggles was terrifying. Fear and anxiety immediately made me imagine the worst-case scenario for my life. Would I ever live a healthy life, have children, and feel like myself again? Could I thrive?

In time, I came to realize that in order to heal, I had to climb the mountain and move beyond fear. I could not have done it without:

Courage. It takes courage to begin and forge the path ahead.

Knowledge. A large part of fear comes from the unknown.

Action. A journey of a thousand miles begins with a single step. Take action.

Persistence. Even when you slip and fall or are fatigued, you brush yourself off, persist, and keep moving forward.

Fear holds back way too many women from thriving. When you allow fear be in control, you are missing out on everything that could be yours. After the three weeks of the 21-Day Plan are finished, keep transcending your fears through courage, knowledge, action, and persistence. Life begins outside of your comfort zone.

Please take the PCOS Diva Symptom Assessment (p. 303) again. Compare your new results with the results of the assessment you took at the beginning of the program. Let these positive results propel you forward to continue to nurture yourself.

Daily Do

Think back to the beginning of the program. When you were prepping for the 21-Day Plan, what were your fears? Were you afraid that you would be hungry all the time? Were you afraid of failure? How did you work through your fears to arrive here at Day 21? What treasures have you discovered along the way? You've scaled the mountain in this program, yet there are many more peaks to climb. How can you continue to move forward with courage, knowledge, action, and persistence?

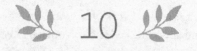

10

Moving Forward

Congratulations, you are a PCOS Diva! The path ahead is full of possibilities. You are a woman with hope. You are in charge of your health and happiness. You take the time and resources to be healthy and fulfilled, and you have seen the benefits of self-care for yourself and those around you. You are an inspiration!

In many ways, you are a different person than you were when you began. You have more energy and a brighter outlook, and you feel stronger. You did that. You made those feelings happen. The good news is that it gets even better. Remember, it takes time to heal. Give yourself a full six months to feel the complete benefits of your lifestyle changes and new habits.

You are already seeing results. From now on, the closer you follow the PCOS Diva lifestyle, the faster you will heal your body, mind, and spirit. Even if you slip a little in the coming weeks and years, you will still progress and thrive. Remember, we are striving for progress, not perfection. I find that living the PCOS Diva lifestyle is self-perpetuating. Once you experience how good feeling good feels, it becomes a healthy addiction, and now it is one you know how to feed.

Your journey has just begun.

What's Next?

Continue to eat a diet that works for you, move every day, maintain your self-care, and above all be kind to yourself. Keep researching and learning about our syndrome, because every PCOS Diva knows that knowledge is power. You have really just begun your PCOS healing journey. Everything you have learned, every habit you have created forms your foundation, but there is so much more you can do.

I encourage you to explore two areas to make your quality of life even better: healing your gut biome and detoxifying your body and environment.

1. Heal your gut, heal your body. The term *microbiome* refers to the bacteria, viruses, fungi, and protozoa that live throughout your body in the gut, nose, throat, mouth, skin, and urogenital tract. These organisms fight pathogens, supply crucial vitamins, and affect weight and metabolism. They are also fundamental to your immune-system function and affect how your genes express themselves. In addition, low bacterial diversity in the gut is associated with leaky gut syndrome, higher body fat, mood disorders, insulin resistance, and inflammation. In fact, an unhealthy microbiome is linked to the development of PCOS.

An imbalance in the gut microbiome can result from a number of factors beginning in utero and extending through birth and breast-feeding and continue to worsen throughout adulthood as a result of the foods and antibiotics we choose. Studies indicate that broad-spectrum antibiotics can alter the gut for up to two years, and conventionally grown and genetically modified crops often contain pesticides and insecticides that disrupt gut bacteria. In this way, even things that are meant to heal or nourish can damage the gut.

You can take steps to heal your gut. Work with your health-care practitioner and consider adding a high-quality probiotic, L-glutamine, deglycyrrhizinated licorice (DGL), or slippery-elm bark to your diet as well as fermented foods and bone-broth soups. Avoid GMO foods, filter your water, and choose organic options when possible. Not only is it possible to heal your own gut and reap the benefits; you can improve the long-term health of future children if you keep your gut bacteria balanced while pregnant and nursing.

2. Detoxify and thrive. Environmental toxins and endocrine disrupting chemicals (EDCs) can undo a lot of the work you are doing to regulate your hormones. In addition, toxins slow down your metabolism and decrease your body's ability to burn fat. You deserve to thrive, but you can't shine your brightest when your body is weighed down with artificial flavors, colors, pesticides, herbicides, and hundreds of other toxins. We put them in our bodies in the form of medications, water, and food, and they are all around us in the environment, from our shampoo to the air we breathe.

Many of the EDCs we encounter very closely resemble our own natural hormones and act as synthetic hormones. Your body's natural estrogen can bind with estrogen receptors, but so can EDCs like bisphenol A (BPA), polychlorinated biphenyls (PCBs), and lots of other chemicals. Found in the products that we use every day, these synthetic hormones mimic or block natural estrogen and testosterone in hormone receptors. As they move throughout your body, they start to turn on or off the hormonal signals that naturally would never have been turned on or off, throwing our systems out of balance.

Many EDCs are "biologically active," meaning they can have an impact, like pharmaceuticals, at very low levels. A lot of people think, "Oh, but it's such a small amount; it won't really matter." Conventional thinking tells us that for something to be toxic, a bigger amount is going to be worse and more dangerous than a smaller amount. And in many cases this *is* true, except when it comes to chemicals that interfere with our endocrine system, in which case *small* amounts may matter more.

Chemicals we're bringing into our homes and our lives, sometimes unwittingly, are silently invading and altering our bodies. Any foreign chemical, whether a pharmaceutical, pesticide, or preservative, can have negative and unintended side effects on our endocrine system. Our bodies detoxify naturally, but can easily get overwhelmed by a tsunami of chemicals that we are exposed to each day, and so those toxins build up. I do the PCOS Diva Sparkle cleanse (PCOSDiva.com

/sparkle) twice a year to ensure that my system stays clear. It is a very gentle, whole-food cleanse that helps my body detoxify itself as it was meant to do. I encourage you to learn more about EDCs and research how to best periodically cleanse your system.

Continue to Upgrade Your Perspective

We hear a lot of doom and gloom about PCOS. Most articles, books, and podcasts seem to focus on the symptoms and potential consequences of PCOS. These should be addressed, I agree, but, you know, there are upsides to PCOS. Instead of lack, look for the abundance. Hear me out.

The knowledge that we are different can be the vehicle that helps us transform our lives and be our truest selves. Taking on the PCOS Diva lifestyle means that you have experienced the wake-up call and taken on the lifestyle upgrades necessary for a healthy life, possibly well before your non-PCOS peers. As a result, you may have prevented much worse symptoms down the road that anyone living an unhealthy lifestyle will experience regardless of a PCOS diagnosis. Without a condition like PCOS, others may suffer the consequences more deeply, because they are not as attuned as we are to the inclinations of our bodies. For example, as women with PCOS, we know we are high-androgen and insulin-resistant, so we know choosing an exercise that will not worsen those hormone levels and that eating a balanced diet full of whole, nutrient-dense foods can help prevent conditions like heart disease and diabetes, for which we are predisposed. We have the advantage of early warning.

PCOS Changed My Life—For the Better

You know my struggle. You know that for a long time I felt that PCOS was robbing me of my life. I felt like a helpless victim of a body that was betraying me. Along my journey, there was a shift. PCOS became my inspiration, not my nemesis. The upgrades I made to my diet, movement, and lifestyle improved my life and the lives of those around me immeasurably.

As I felt better and changed my behaviors, my family noticed the improvement and began to make changes themselves. My doctor started referring PCOS patients to me. I was able to help those women, and word spread. Soon PCOS Diva was born, and now, years later, thousands of women have embraced the PCOS Diva lifestyle and are thriving with PCOS.

Had I continued to let PCOS happen to me, had I failed to learn to work with my body, had I remained a victim, these women may never have found their personal keys to healing and hundreds of babies may not exist!

Most important, PCOS and my healing journey opened my eyes to my own potential and possibility. I became empowered to find answers and feel and do good. I make choices that benefit my health and, so, benefit others. The old saying that you can't pour from an empty cup is true.

The Upsides of PCOS

Believe it or not, PCOS can offer some other physical benefits. One of the women who has been instrumental in changing *my* view of PCOS is Nancy Dunne, a naturopathic physician in Missoula, Montana. Considered a pioneer in the PCOS world, Dunne tells her PCOS patients during consultations all about the *advantages* of being a high-androgen insulin-resistant woman. That's right—advantages, not disadvantages. Yes, we should endeavor to heal our bodies, but our unique PCOS characteristics offer some unexpected benefits.

Women with PCOS remain fertile longer. Data suggest women with PCOS *do* have a harder time conceiving than women without the condition, but they remain fertile longer. Several studies have hinted at this likelihood, but some findings include the fact that women with PCOS may have a greater egg reserve than women without PCOS, because they ovulate less regularly and their ovaries start out with denser follicles at primary stages compared with "normal" ovaries.

Think of delayed fertility as a chance not to face familial and child-rearing obligations as early in life as some of our peers without PCOS, and thus an opportunity to gain maturity and get our affairs in order. View PCOS as a chance to focus on *you* before you grow your family.

Women with PCOS have a higher threshold for pain. According to a 2016 study, concentration of plasma beta-endorphin levels can increase the pressure pain threshold (PPT), and in this study researchers measured those markers in forty-eight lean women with PCOS and thirty-eight controls. They found that the beta-endorphin serum level and PPT were higher in the lean PCOS group than in the controls.

Women with PCOS are made to survive. A 2011 report lists various studies detailing the potential evolutionary advantage of women with PCOS. It explains that women with this disorder may have a "thrifty genotype" that made them more likely to survive than women without PCOS during times of food deprivation and less likely to expend as much energy.

Women with PCOS may have stronger bones. According to a 2000 analysis, various studies link high androgen levels to greater bone mass density, leaving women with PCOS (who are inherently high-androgen) at a lower risk of osteoporosis.

Women with PCOS have superior visual spatial skills. According to a 2013 study, researchers found that women with PCOS scored "significantly higher on a mental rotation task than a female control group." Their higher testosterone levels may be the reason why, as previous studies have linked the elevated hormone to greater performance of three-dimensional mental rotation tasks.

Women with PCOS have more muscle strength. A 2014 study examined forty women with PCOS and forty without the condition and drew a link between high androgen levels in the PCOS group to greater muscle strength in various exercises, including bicep curls, handgrip strength tests, and bench presses.

Women with high testosterone and elevated cortisol levels make better leaders. Research suggests that feedback networks between the brain and hormones work against each other to regulate dominant and competitive behaviors. As a result, women with high testosterone and cortisol may be more assertive.

Women with high testosterone take riskier jobs. In 2009, researchers surveyed five hundred male and female MBA students at the University of Chicago. When asked whether they would take a job that had a guaranteed monetary reward or a risky lottery with a bigger potential payout, women with more testosterone showed a greater likelihood of taking the risk, but the same was not true for men.

Although PCOS research is emerging every month as more patients and doctors become aware of this condition, what we know now is that there is a lot to be grateful for with PCOS.

Moving Forward with Gratitude

Throughout the plan, I have encouraged you to list what you are grateful for every morning and every night. If there is only one "aha" moment that you take away from this experience, let it be gratitude. Going forward, approach life from a place of abundance, not a place of lack. Live each day with gratitude for all you have and your PCOS Diva journey, which has helped you to discover who you really are: healthier, stronger, more hopeful, abundant, compassionate, and resilient. *Shifting your perspective to a place of gratitude and abundance is the ultimate secret to thriving with PCOS.*

Ultimately, if you want more health, happiness, joy, and energy in your life, you must cultivate gratitude. Gratitude moves us from limitation, lack, and fear to abundance, health, and love.

Final Thoughts

As you move forward in your PCOS Diva journey, I hope you have come to realize that this condition is not a life sentence to misery or a less-than life. As a PCOS Diva, you have hope, promise, and potential! You can and will *thrive* and live an *abundant, vibrant* life—your *best* life.

Sometimes that means pressing yourself through the fear and anxiety of an opportunity to try something new. When this happens, I hope that you muster up the courage of your PCOS Diva and rocket-launch yourself into new possibilities. Together, your newfound courage, hope, and gratitude give you personal power beyond belief.

I am grateful that I get to do what I love every day—and that is to show women like myself that they can thrive with PCOS, not despite it. You are grateful, empowered, and in control again. Be hopeful. I promise, the more you focus on the good in your life, the more good you will have in your life. Live gratefully and abundantly, PCOS Diva!

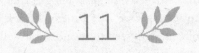

Recipes

This collection of recipes is just the starting point for your food journey. You will soon discover that healthy and healing food is delicious and satisfying. Every recipe I created for the Healing PCOS 21-Day Plan is family- and friend-tested and fits the PCOS Diva guidelines. That means they are all gluten and processed soy free, low dairy, and whole-foods based.

Keep in mind, this is an individualized plan; everybody is different. Maybe you need more protein and less starch. Maybe you can't tolerate oats. Listen to your body and adjust using the guidelines covered in Chapter 4. Try making these dishes according the recipe the first time; then get creative and make them your own. Once you learn your body's rhythm, developing menus becomes a snap.

Sustainability is the goal of eating like a PCOS Diva. Find what works for you in this collection and automate it. Always keep the basic items stocked (supplement powders, nondairy milk, eggs, and frozen fruit, for example). If you can make a quick meal or snack without having to give it a ton of thought, that healthy meal becomes a healthy habit that is easy to maintain. The most "perfect" recipe in the world won't help you if you never have the time or the exotic ingredients on hand to make it. Keep it simple. Be kind to yourself; *feel and taste the difference!*

These recipes are designed to help wean you off of sugar-laden sweet foods and satisfy you with naturally sweet foods like fruits or options sweetened with a little maple syrup or raw honey. This transition will take time. You may still have sugar cravings. You will want to add more sweetener to some recipes. Be patient. It took a while for your taste buds to become desensitized to sugar, and it will take time to re-sensitize them to appreciate the flavors and natural sweetness of whole foods. As always, I encourage you to experiment and find a whole-food sweetener that works for you, or just eliminate the sweetener entirely from the recipe. It's up to you!

You will quickly notice the theme of *layering*. Being a PCOS Diva is not about deprivation and denial. Our meals shouldn't all taste like lettuce. *Layer ingredients and flavors to assure that you are getting both the nutrients you need and the flavor you desire!*

Finally, let your time in the kitchen be a "meditation moment" whenever possible. Be mindful while you chop, peel, and sauté. For more recipe ideas, download the PCOS Diva Seasonal Meal Plans and slow cooker guide available at PCOSDiva.com/meal-plans.

Now, get cooking!

Breakfast

Let's be real. No one has the time or inclination to pull out a cookbook every morning and whip up an elaborate breakfast. It is important to start your day off on the right foot, but there is a reason people resort to cereal—it's easy. The Healing PCOS 21-Day Plan has a system to help you consistently have satisfying breakfasts that will get you through the morning without a lot of hassle and help you build a sustainable habit. *The trick is to find a few simple favorites that work for you and always stock the basic ingredients.*

I encourage you to try all of these recipes and journal how you feel after you eat them, noting how long your energy lasts, when you next feel hungry, and any other physical or emotional reactions you experience. Then pick the ones that are best for *you*. Once you have chosen, making a healthy breakfast becomes as routine as brushing your teeth.

I have found that smoothies satisfy and energize me on most days, yet when the weather turns frigid, as it does in January and February where I live, I reach for my Super-Seed Quick Oats. In my pre–PCOS Diva days, I would enjoy waffles, muffins, and pancakes almost every day of the week. Filled with white flour and processed sugar, these breakfast items did nothing to help balance blood sugar or nourish my body for the day ahead. I must admit, I do still enjoy a muffin or plate of pancakes, but I think of them as a sweet-treat indulgence. I limit myself to enjoying them on the weekend, and I make a PCOS Diva version. I like to stick with more nutrient-rich breakfasts during the week and enjoy these occasionally on the weekend.

SMOOTHIES

Making smoothies couldn't be easier. They take 1 minute to whip up and you can drink them on the go. Be sure to keep smoothie ingredients stocked in your pantry, refrigerator, and freezer.

7-Layer Smoothie

Makes 1 serving

This basic smoothie recipe is very flexible, with lots of options. Change the flavors with the season or your mood by using different kinds of fruit.

1st Layer: Unsweetened Nondairy Liquid Base

You can make your own homemade nut milks or purchase unsweetened nonsoy, nondairy milks at the grocery store. The amount of liquid in your smoothie will determine the consistency. Less liquid will make for a thicker smoothie, while more liquid will give you a thinner drink. I like to use 1 cup of nondairy milk and add ice or water if needed.

1 cup of any of the following (unsweetened):
- Coconut milk
- Hemp milk
- Almond milk
- Cashew milk

- Green tea
- Chai tea
- Coconut water

2nd Layer: Protein Powder

1 scoop or serving PCOS Diva Power Protein or Power Vegan Protein,
vanilla or chocolate (or similar protein powder)

3rd Layer: Fruit and Greens

Use high-glycemic tropical fruits or melons infrequently and keep the portion
size small. I leave the skins on fruit for extra nutrients.

Any of the following (but do not exceed 1 cup fruit maximum):
- ½ to 1 cup berries
- 1 medium apple, cored and chopped
- 1 medium pear, cored and chopped
- 2 kiwis, peeled and chopped
- ½ to 1 cup stone fruit, pitted and chopped (peaches, plums, cherries,
  nectarines, apricots)
- ½ cup pumpkin puree
- ½ small banana
- ¼ cup pineapple or mango, peeled and chopped

½ cup of any of the following fresh greens, ribs removed:
- Dandelion greens
- Spinach
- Kale
- Romaine
- Chard
- Beet greens

4th Layer: Healthy Fat

1 tablespoon of any of the following:
- Coconut manna
- Virgin coconut oil
- MCT oil
- Nut or seed butter

Or ¼ to ½ avocado

5th Layer: Fiber

If you are not currently eating lots of fiber, ramp up slowly. Start by adding
just a little fiber to your smoothies.

1 tablespoon of any of the following:
- PCOS Diva Power Fiber (or similar fiber powder;
  start with 2 teaspoons and use more if tolerated)
- Unsweetened coconut flakes
- Coconut flour
- Hemp seeds
- Chia seeds
- Ground flaxseed

6th Layer: Flavoring

Any of the following to taste:
- Pure extract (vanilla, lemon, almond, coconut, maple,
  peppermint; I suggest ¼ to ½ teaspoon)
- Vanilla powder
- Raw cacao
- Fresh mint
- Cacao nibs
- Fresh ginger
- Spices (ground nutmeg, cloves, cardamom, cinnamon,
  ginger, cayenne, Pumpkin Pie Spice [p. 285])
- Lemon or lime zest
- Pink Himalayan salt

7th Layer: Nutrient Boost

Any or all of the following:
- ½ teaspoon matcha tea powder
- ½-inch piece fresh turmeric root, grated, or ½ teaspoon powder
- 1 tablespoon PCOS Diva Power Greens (or similar greens powder)
- 1 tablespoon PCOS Diva Power Reds (or similar reds powder)
- 1 teaspoon PCOS Diva Super Magnesium (or similar magnesium powder)
- 2000 mg myo-inositol powder (or one packet of Ovasitol)
- 500 mg L-glutamine powder

Blend all of the ingredients in a high-speed blender until smooth. Add ice or water until it reaches the desired consistency.

Apple Pie Smoothie

Makes 1 serving
- 1 cup unsweetened almond milk
- 1 scoop PCOS Diva Power Protein, vanilla flavor (or similar protein powder)
- 1 medium apple, cored and chopped

1 handful baby spinach
2 teaspoons PCOS Diva Fiber Powder (or similar fiber powder)
1 tablespoon almond butter
½ teaspoon pure vanilla extract
½ teaspoon ground cinnamon
¼ teaspoon freshly grated nutmeg
1 tablespoon PCOS Diva Power Greens (or similar greens powder)

Blend all of the ingredients in a high-speed blender until smooth. Add ice or water until it reaches the desired consistency.

Ginger Peach Smoothie

Makes 1 serving

1 cup unsweetened coconut milk
1 scoop PCOS Diva Power Vegan Protein, vanilla flavor
    (or similar protein powder)
½ cup frozen peaches
1 handful kale, ribs removed, roughly chopped
1 tablespoon MCT oil
1 tablespoon ground flaxseed
1 tablespoon grated fresh ginger (use less if you like it less zippy)
½ teaspoon pure vanilla extract
½ teaspoon ground cinnamon
Dash of ground cardamom (optional)
½ teaspoon matcha tea powder

Blend all of the ingredients in a high-speed blender until smooth. Add ice or water until it reaches the desired consistency.

Chocolate Cherry-Berry Smoothie

Makes 1 serving

1 cup unsweetened cashew milk
1 scoop PCOS Diva Power Protein, chocolate (or similar protein powder)
½ cup frozen blackberries
½ cup frozen cherries
3 large romaine leaves
¼ avocado
1 tablespoon hemp seeds
½ teaspoon pure vanilla extract
1 tablespoon raw cacao powder

Blend all of the ingredients in a high-speed blender until smooth. Add ice or water until it reaches the desired consistency.

CHIA PUDDING

Chia seeds are a complete protein source and contain lots of omega–3 fatty acids and fiber. They will soak up any liquid and swell to ten times their weight to create a gel that is similar in consistency to a tapioca pudding. Chia pudding is made by combining chia seeds with nondairy milk, sweeteners, flavorings, and various nutritional boosts and leaving it in the refrigerator overnight. In the morning, you can layer the pudding with fruit, nuts, seeds, and other toppings for a quick and yummy breakfast. As with smoothies, there are lots of flavor combinations to keep you free from breakfast boredom.

Be sure to use whole chia seeds and not ground; ground seeds do not congeal as well. Play with the ratio of chia seeds to liquid to find a consistency that you enjoy.

Chia Pudding Parfait

Makes 1 serving

The chia pudding (layers 1 through 5) for this breakfast *must be prepared at least 2 hours ahead* (12 hours would be best) and will last two to three days in the refrigerator.

1st Layer: Unsweetened Nondairy Milk

1 cup of any of the following:
- Coconut milk
- Hemp milk
- Almond milk
- Cashew milk

2nd Layer: Whole Chia Seeds

3 to 4 tablespoons white or black chia seeds

3rd Layer: Sweetener (optional)

Liquid natural sweeteners like maple syrup and honey are the easiest to blend in your pudding. If you choose honey, you may need to heat it slightly so that it incorporates well.

1 to 2 teaspoons of any of the following:
- Maple syrup
- Raw honey
- Coconut nectar

4th Layer: Flavoring

Any of the following to taste:
- Lemon or lime zest
- Spices (ground nutmeg, cloves, cardamom, cinnamon, ginger, Pumpkin Pie Spice [p. 285])
- Pure extract (vanilla, lemon, almond, coconut, maple, peppermint; I suggest ¼ to ½ teaspoon)

5th Layer: Nutrient Boost (optional)

1 tablespoon of any of the following:
- Nut or seed butter
- Virgin coconut oil or manna
- Cacao powder
- Collagen powder
- Matcha powder (½ teaspoon)

6th Layer: Toppings

Raw or Cooked Fruit

One of any of the following:
- ½ cup berries (you can also macerate the berries for at least 30 minutes with a bit of freshly squeezed lemon juice and 1 teaspoon of coconut sugar to make a sauce)
- ½ medium apple, cored and chopped
- ½ medium pear, cored and chopped
- 2 kiwis, peeled and chopped
- ½ cup stone fruit, pitted and chopped (peaches, plums, cherries, nectarines, apricots)
- ¼ cup mango or pineapple, peeled and chopped
- ¼ cup banana, chopped
- ¼ cup pomegranate arils
- ⅓ cup sliced fresh figs
- ¼ cup unsweetened applesauce

- ¼ cup pumpkin puree
- ⅓ cup Stewed Spiced Fruit (p. 288; apples, pears, or peaches)

Dry Toppings

1 tablespoon (maximum) dried fruit (cranberries, blueberries, strawberries, currants, goji berries, apricots)
1 or more tablespoons of any of the following:
- Chopped or sliced nuts
- Sunflower seeds, pepitas, or hemp seeds
- Cacao nibs
- Unsweetened coconut

Pour layers 1 through 4 or 5 (see Note, just below) into a pint-size Mason jar, seal tightly, shake vigorously, and let it sit for 30 minutes. Shake the jar again and then set it in the refrigerator overnight to thicken. In the morning, dish out the pudding and add toppings.

Note: If you incorporate the 5th layer, first warm the milk in a small saucepan over medium heat and stir in the nutrient boost. Remove the milk from the heat and pour it into the jar. Then add the chia seeds, sweetener, and flavoring to the warmed milk. The heating helps to incorporate the nutrient boost.

Chocolate-Almond-Strawberry Chia Pudding

Makes 1 serving

1 cup unsweetened coconut milk
1 tablespoon cacao powder
2 to 3 tablespoons chia seeds
2 to 3 teaspoons honey
½ teaspoon pure almond extract
2 tablespoons hemp seeds
2 tablespoons sliced almonds
½ cup sliced strawberries, macerated with a squeeze of lemon juice and 1 teaspoon coconut sugar

In a small saucepan over medium heat, warm the milk and cacao powder. Remove the cacao mixture from the heat and pour it into a pint-size Mason jar. Add the chia seeds, honey, and almond extract. Seal the jar tightly, shake vigorously, and let sit for 30 minutes. Shake the jar again and then set it in the refrigerator overnight to thicken.

To serve, top with hemp seeds, sliced almonds, and macerated strawberries.

OATS

I love hot oatmeal for breakfast on dark, cold winter mornings. Oats are hearty and fill me up for hours. Grain-based porridges may not work for some PCOS Divas. Start by trying my Super-Seed Quick Oats. If they work for you, try my Slow-Cooker Steel-Cut Oats and Overnight Blueberry Buckle Steel-Cut Oats.

Cooking your oats overnight in a slow cooker is a great option. However, I suggest that you do a trial run during the day when you are home in order to determine how long your oats will need to cook. Every slow cooker is different. I cook mine for 8 hours on low for perfect oatmeal. I turn it on before bed, and it is warm and ready when I get up.

Super-Seed Quick Oats

Makes 1 serving

1st Layer: Unsweetened Nondairy Milk

1 cup of any of the following:
- Coconut milk
- Hemp milk
- Almond milk
- Cashew milk

2nd Layer: Sweetener

1 to 2 teaspoons of any of the following:
- Maple syrup
- Raw honey
- Coconut nectar
- Coconut sugar

3rd Layer: Fat

1 tablespoon of any of the following:
- Grass-fed butter
- Grass-fed ghee
- Virgin coconut oil
- Nut butter

4th Layer: Flavoring

Any of the following to taste:
- Pure extract (vanilla, lemon, almond, coconut, maple;
  I suggest ¼ to ½ teaspoon)
- Sea salt
- Spices (ground nutmeg, cloves, cardamom, cinnamon, ginger,
  Pumpkin Pie Spice [p. 285])

5th Layer: Oats

½ cup gluten-free old-fashioned rolled oats

6th Layer: Seeds

1 tablespoon of *each* of the following:
- Chia seeds
- Ground flaxseed
- Pepitas
- Sunflower seeds

—————————————— Time-Saving Tip ——————————————

Premix a large batch of layers 5 and 6. Thoroughly combine the oats
and seeds and store in an airtight container. Use a heaping ½ cup when
measuring a serving size.

7th Layer: Protein Powder (optional)

½ scoop or serving PCOS Diva Power Protein or Power Vegan Protein, vanilla
or chocolate (or similar protein powder)

8th Layer: Toppings (optional)

Any of the Chia Pudding Parfait toppings (pp. 232–33)

In a small saucepan over medium-low heat, warm the milk and sweetener,
stirring occasionally, until the milk is hot and steamy. Add the fat. When it has
melted, add the flavorings. Remove from the heat.

In a pint-size Mason jar, layer the oats, seeds, and protein powder. Pour
the hot milk over the oat mixture and stir to combine. Cover the jar with a lid
and let it sit for 10 minutes to thicken. Remove the lid, stir, and add desired
toppings.

Apple Cobbler Super-Seed Quick Oats

Makes 1 serving

- 1 cup unsweetened almond milk
- 2 teaspoons maple syrup
- 1 tablespoon grass-fed butter
- ¼ teaspoon pure vanilla extract
- ½ teaspoon ground cinnamon
- Pinch freshly grated nutmeg
- Pinch ground cloves
- Pinch sea salt
- ½ cup gluten-free old-fashioned rolled oats
- 1 tablespoon chia seeds
- 1 tablespoon ground flaxseed
- 1 tablespoon pepitas
- 1 tablespoon sunflower seeds
- ¼ cup unsweetened applesauce
- 2 tablespoons toasted coarsely chopped pecans
- 1 tablespoon dried cranberries

In a small saucepan over medium-low heat, warm the milk and maple syrup, stirring occasionally, until the milk is hot and steamy. Add the butter, stirring until melted, and then add the vanilla, cinnamon, nutmeg, cloves, and salt. Remove from the heat.

In a pint-size Mason jar, layer the oats, chia seeds, flaxseed, pepitas, and sunflower seeds. Pour the hot milk over the oat mixture and stir to combine. Cover the jar with a lid and let it sit 10 minutes to thicken. Remove the lid and stir in the applesauce, pecans, and cranberries.

Slow-Cooker Steel-Cut Oats

Makes 4 servings

As an alternative to my Super-Seed Quick Oats, I love steel-cut oats for breakfast. They are loaded with fiber, which is key for removing toxins and excess hormones from your body. Also referred to as Irish or Scottish oats, this type of oatmeal is processed by chopping the whole oat groat into several pieces rather than rolling it. Steel-cut oats must be cooked much longer than rolled oats. So if you are short on time in the morning, the oats can be cooked at the beginning of the week and placed in an airtight container in the refrigerator. Each day scoop out a portion, add some nondairy milk, and reheat.

1st Layer: Oats

1 cup gluten-free steel-cut oats

2nd Layer: Water

4 cups filtered water

3rd Layer: Sweetener

3 tablespoons of any of the following:
- Maple syrup
- Raw honey
- Coconut nectar
- Coconut sugar

4th Layer: Flavoring

Any of the following:
- 1 to 2 teaspoons pure extract (vanilla, almond, coconut, maple)
- ½ teaspoon sea salt
- Spices to taste (ground nutmeg, cloves, cardamom, cinnamon, ginger, Pumpkin Pie Spice [p. 285])

5th Layer: Fat

3 tablespoons of any of the following:
- Grass-fed butter
- Grass-fed ghee
- Virgin coconut oil
- Nut butter

6th Layer: Protein Powder (optional)

1 scoop or serving of PCOS Diva Power Protein or Power Vegan Protein, vanilla or chocolate (or similar protein powder)

7th Layer: Toppings

Any of the Chia Pudding Parfait toppings (pp. 232–33)

8th Layer: Unsweetened Nondairy Milk

½ cup of any of the following:
- Coconut milk
- Hemp milk
- Almond milk
- Cashew milk

Place the first 4 layers in a slow cooker and cook on low for 8 hours or overnight. Before serving, stir in layers 5 through 8.

Overnight Blueberry Buckle Steel-Cut Oats

Makes 4 servings

    1 cup gluten-free steel-cut oats
    4 cups water
    3 tablespoons raw honey
    2 teaspoons pure vanilla extract
    2 teaspoons ground cinnamon
    ½ teaspoon sea salt
    3 tablespoons virgin coconut oil
    1 scoop PCOS Diva Power Protein, vanilla (or similar protein powder)
    ¼ cup dried apricots, chopped
    2 cups fresh blueberries
    ⅓ cup walnuts, chopped
    ½ cup unsweetened almond milk

In a slow cooker, layer the oats through the salt and cook on low for 8 hours or overnight. To serve, stir in coconut oil, protein powder, apricots, blueberries, walnuts, and milk until well combined.

EGGS

Eggs are an excellent breakfast choice for many women with PCOS, but a large number of people are sensitive to eggs. It is an important part of your PCOS Diva health journey to be tested for food sensitivities. If you are continually eating a food that you are sensitive to, it will cause more inflammation.

I like to combine eggs with veggies and greens in the morning. For a very hearty, savory breakfast, lunch, or even dinner, top your oats with eggs. Think Garlicky Greens (p. 278), bacon, and a poached egg on top of your Super-Seed Quick Oats.

Avocado, Egg, and Arugula Rice-Cake Breakfast Toast

Makes 1 serving

There are many variations on avocado breakfast toast. I like to use a brown-rice cake instead of a slice of gluten-free toast. You can cook your egg any way you please: poached, fried, scrambled, or soft-boiled. You can also add or replace the egg with smoked salmon, bacon, or slices of turkey. Don't skip the vegetables.

- ½ avocado
- 2 teaspoons olive-oil mayonnaise
- Sea salt to taste
- 1 brown-rice cake
- 1 large hard-boiled organic, free-range egg, sliced
- ½ cup baby spinach leaves
- ⅓ cup arugula
- ½ medium tomato, sliced
- 2 fresh basil leaves, shredded
- 2 green onions, chopped

Mash the avocado with the mayonnaise and salt. Spread the mixture on the rice cake. Layer egg slices, spinach leaves, arugula, tomato, basil, and green onions on top.

Spinach, Tomato, and Basil Egg Scramble

Makes 2 servings

An egg scramble is a quick and easy way to get some veggies in the morning. This is my favorite combination, but you can use any variety of veggies for a morning scramble. Depending on how I feel, I may sauté the spinach with the tomatoes or top it with raw baby spinach chiffonade.

- 1 teaspoon virgin coconut oil
- 1 cup baby spinach leaves
- ½ large fresh tomato, seeded and diced
- 2 fresh basil leaves, finely shredded
- 1 small clove garlic, minced
- 2 large organic, free-range eggs, beaten
- Sea salt and freshly ground black pepper to taste

In a skillet over medium heat, heat the oil. Add the spinach, diced tomatoes, basil, and garlic and sauté for 2 minutes. Add the beaten eggs and cook, stirring occasionally to cook the eggs through, about 5 minutes. Season with salt and pepper.

Sausage, Asparagus, and Egg Muffin Cups

Makes 6 servings

Make a batch of these muffin cups on Sunday, and you'll have breakfast for most of your week. They last four days in the refrigerator. These can also be frozen and reheated for a quick breakfast on the run. Again, experiment with lots of different flavor combinations. Just be sure to add your veggies!

    1 tablespoon avocado oil
    1 cup chopped red pepper
    1 cup chopped yellow pepper
    1 cup chopped onion
    6 links (about 4 ounces) turkey or chicken breakfast sausage
        (I like Applegate Farms Chicken and Sage)
    1 cup chopped asparagus (woody stem ends removed)
    2 cloves garlic, minced
    8 large organic, free-range eggs
    ½ teaspoon sea salt
    ¼ teaspoon freshly ground black pepper

Preheat the oven to 350°F. Line 12 standard-size muffin cups with parchment cupcake liners. Heat the oil in a large skillet over medium heat. Add the peppers, onion, and sausage. As the sausage begins to cook, break it up into small bite-size pieces. Sauté for 5 minutes and then add the asparagus and sauté for an additional 3 minutes until tender. Add the garlic, stir to combine, and remove from the heat.

In a large mixing bowl, beat the eggs and season with salt and pepper. Stir in the cooked meat and veggies. Pour the egg mixture into the prepared muffin cups and bake for 15 to 20 minutes, until the eggs are set to the touch.

PROTEIN BARS

Make a batch or two of protein bars to keep on hand in the freezer. They defrost very quickly. There is nothing faster than grabbing a bar from your freezer on your way out the door on a frenzied morning. Although these bars aren't my ideal breakfast, because my body feels better with smoothies or oats, they are perfect in a pinch and double for a great afternoon snack as well. These gluten-free, vegan, and mostly raw bars are just the thing for breakfast-evading PCOS Divas.

Pumpkin Spice Protein Bars

Makes 12 bars

1½ cups gluten-free old-fashioned rolled oats
1 cup PCOS Diva Power Protein, vanilla flavored (or similar protein powder)
½ cup raisins
½ cup chopped walnuts
¼ cup pepitas
2 tablespoons ground flaxseed
2 tablespoons chia seeds
1 tablespoon Pumpkin Pie Spice (p. 285)
½ teaspoon sea salt
½ cup canned pumpkin (not pumpkin pie filling)
½ cup unsalted almond butter
⅓ cup maple syrup
1 teaspoon pure vanilla extract
¼ cup virgin coconut oil, melted (optional)
½ cup flaked unsweetened coconut (optional)

In a large bowl, combine the oats, protein powder, raisins, walnuts, pepitas, flaxseed, chia seeds, Pumpkin Pie Spice, and sea salt. In a small bowl, combine the canned pumpkin, almond butter, maple syrup, and vanilla extract. If adding coconut oil, melt it over very low heat and then add it to the wet mixture. Fold the wet mixture into the dry and stir in the coconut flakes (if using).

Spread the mixture into an 8 × 8-inch baking pan lined with parchment paper. Press firmly until flat. Freeze or refrigerate until just set. Cut into 12 granola-style bars. Wrap bars individually and store in the freezer for a grab-and-go breakfast or snack. Store in the freezer for up to one month.

Chocolate Mint Protein Bars

Makes 12 bars

1½ cups gluten-free old-fashioned rolled oats
½ cup raw almonds, finely chopped
½ cup raw walnuts, finely chopped
1 cup PCOS Diva Power Protein, chocolate (or similar protein powder)
⅓ cup plus 1 tablespoon finely ground almond flour
¼ cup plus 1 tablespoon raw cacao powder
2 tablespoons hemp seeds
1 tablespoon chia seeds
½ cup unsweetened applesauce
2 tablespoons maple syrup
1 teaspoon pure peppermint extract
36 chocolate chips (optional; I like Ghirardelli 60 percent cacao chips)

Grind the gluten-free oats in high-speed blender or food processor until they form a coarse flour. Place the flour in a large bowl. Add the nuts, protein powder, almond flour, cacao powder, hemp seeds, and chia seeds. In a small bowl, combine the applesauce, maple syrup, and peppermint extract. Fold the applesauce mixture into the oat-flour mixture. Combine well. The mixture will be sticky.

Spread the mixture into an 8 × 8-inch baking pan lined with parchment paper. If using chocolate chips, sprinkle on top of the bars and press firmly until the surface is flat. Freeze or refrigerate until just set. Cut into 12 granola-style bars. Wrap the bars individually and store in the freezer for a grab-and-go breakfast or snack. Store in the freezer for up to one month.

SPECIAL SUNDAY MORNING TREATS

Who doesn't love a leisurely Sunday morning breakfast of homemade muffins, scones, pancakes, or waffles? Yet a typical white-flour baked good can send your blood sugar soaring. You can have an occasional muffin and eat it too with my take on these cozy breakfast treats. Sunday breakfasts are an opportunity to mindfully indulge. During the week, stick with smoothies, chia puddings, oatmeal, and eggs. Treat pancakes, waffles, and muffins like a sweet-treat indulgence. Make a PCOS Diva version so that you can indulge and still feel terrific. They all freeze well.

Harvest Muffins

Makes 12 muffins

Coconut-oil cooking spray
½ cup canned pumpkin
2 large organic, free-range eggs, lightly beaten
¼ cup maple syrup or raw honey
2 tablespoons virgin coconut oil
1 teaspoon pure vanilla extract
¼ cup unsweetened applesauce
1 apple, cored and grated
2 cups finely ground almond flour
½ cup ground flaxseed
1 teaspoon baking powder
1 tablespoon apple pie spice (or a mix of ground cinnamon,
    nutmeg, cloves, and allspice)
¼ cup chopped walnuts or pecans
¼ cup dried cranberries
¼ cup unsweetened coconut flakes

Preheat the oven to 350°F. Coat 12 standard-size muffin cups with coconut-oil cooking spray.

In a large bowl, combine the pumpkin, eggs, maple syrup or honey, coconut oil, vanilla extract, applesauce, and grated apple. In a separate bowl, combine the almond flour, flaxseed, baking powder, and apple pie spice. Add the dry mixture to the wet mixture until just combined. Fold in the nuts, cranberries, and coconut.

Spoon the batter (it will be thick) equally into the muffin cups. Bake for 30 to 35 minutes, until the tops of the muffins are brown and firm and a toothpick inserted comes out clean. If you like a drier muffin, you may need to bake them a bit longer. Cool on a baking rack.

Fruit Scones

Makes 8 scones

This recipe works with a variety of berries, such as blueberries, raspberries, blackberries, or chopped strawberries. You can also try chopped peaches, plums, mango, or even cherries. Alternatively, use almond extract instead of vanilla.

2 cups finely ground almond flour
½ cup coconut flour

¼ cup coconut sugar
½ teaspoon sea salt
½ teaspoon baking soda
1 teaspoon pure vanilla extract
2 large organic, free-range eggs, lightly beaten
¼ cup grass-fed butter, melted
½ cup chopped fresh fruit

Preheat the oven to 350°F. In a large mixing bowl, combine the almond flour, coconut flour, coconut sugar, salt, and baking soda. In a smaller bowl, combine the extract, eggs, and melted butter. Mix the wet ingredients into the dry and fold in the fruit. Gather the dough to form a ball and turn it out onto a baking sheet lined with parchment paper. Pat the dough into a disk about 1 inch thick. Cut into 8 wedges and separate. Bake until lightly browned, about 15 minutes.

Waffles with Coconut Cream and Strawberries

Makes 6 4-inch-square waffles

Waffles

1 cup gluten-free all-purpose flour
½ cup coconut flour
½ cup finely ground almond flour
1 tablespoon baking powder
½ teaspoon baking soda
½ teaspoon sea salt
2 tablespoons coconut sugar
1½ cups unsweetened coconut milk
1 teaspoon pure vanilla extract
2 large organic, free-range eggs, separated
¼ cup grass-fed butter, melted
Coconut-oil cooking spray

Coconut Cream

1 (13.5-ounce) can full-fat coconut milk, well chilled
   (I like to leave it in the refrigerator overnight)
2 tablespoons maple syrup
1 tablespoon arrowroot powder
1 teaspoon pure vanilla extract

For Serving

2 cups sliced strawberries
Freshly grated nutmeg

For the waffles: Heat a waffle iron. In a mixing bowl, combine the all-purpose flour, coconut flour, almond flour, baking powder, baking soda, salt, and coconut sugar until well combined. In smaller bowl, mix the coconut milk, vanilla, egg yolks, and butter. In another small bowl, beat the egg whites until stiff peaks form. Add the wet ingredients to the dry and whisk together until slightly lumpy. Fold in the egg whites. Coat the heated waffle iron with coconut-oil spray, pour 1/3 cup batter for each waffle into the waffle iron, and cook until brown and crispy, 6 to 7 minutes.

For the coconut cream: Open the well-chilled can of coconut milk and scoop out the solid cream that has risen to the top into a bowl. Discard the coconut water. With an electric hand mixer, whip the cream, maple syrup, arrowroot, and vanilla extract to the desired consistency.

To serve, top each waffle with 1/3 cup sliced strawberries, 2 to 3 tablespoons coconut cream, and a sprinkle of freshly grated nutmeg.

Variations: For Chocolate Waffles, add ¼ cup of raw cacao powder to the batter. For Fall Waffles, add pumpkin pie spice (p. 285) or apple pie spice and a couple of tablespoons dried cranberries and finely chopped walnuts.

Lemon Poppy-Seed Pancakes

Makes 4 servings; 1 serving: 2 pancakes

1 cup gluten-free all-purpose flour
½ cup finely ground almond flour
¼ cup PCOS Diva Power Protein, vanilla (or similar protein powder)
2 teaspoons baking powder
¼ teaspoon sea salt
1 large organic, free-range egg, lightly beaten
1 tablespoon virgin coconut oil, melted
1 teaspoon pure lemon extract
1 cup unsweetened almond milk
2 tablespoons poppy seeds
Zest of 1 lemon
Coconut-oil cooking spray
2 cups raspberries

In a medium bowl, mix together the flour, almond flour, protein powder, baking powder, and salt. In smaller bowl, combine the egg, coconut oil, extract, and almond milk. Add the wet mixture to the dry mixture and stir until just blended. Stir in the poppy seeds and lemon zest.

Coat a griddle or nonstick skillet with coconut-oil spray and heat over medium heat. Ladle about ¼ cup of the batter onto the griddle to make a pancake (you should be able to fit two or three on a large griddle). Cook the pancakes until you begin to see bubbles coming through the batter. Flip gently, and cook until golden brown. Serve with fresh raspberries.

Lunch

Lunch is the easiest meal to automate. Typically, PCOS Divas try to make an extra serving or two of dinner that can be used for lunch the next day. Not only does it make lunch easy, but you will have a meal that you actually look forward to enjoying on your lunch break and one you will finish feeling great. Just watch out for coworkers who might be tempted to steal your gorgeous lunches!

We also love Salads in a Jar. The layering technique takes the hassle out of creating and packing a salad. Get creative with your salad. It doesn't have to be the same ol' iceberg lettuce, cuke, and tomato salad you may have grown up with. In the spring and summer, when farm-fresh greens are in abundance, I almost always have a salad with either protein or roasted/grilled veggies left over from dinner the night before. I also love bean spreads and dips with the same proteins or veggies.

Lunches should follow the proportions on the PCOS Diva Plate. Keep your ratios around ¼ protein, ¼ starchy/root veggies or grains, and ½ leafy greens and nonstarchy veggies. Add a generous splash of healthy fat, and you're ready to go!

A Note About Salad Dressings: Women with PCOS have to be very careful about the oils we put in our bodies. Store-bought salad dressings almost always contain oils we are trying to avoid, such as soybean oil. Making your own salad dressings is very simple and quick. Try to get in the habit of making a batch to use throughout your week. There are countless combinations and flavors you can use, and many dressings can double as marinades. I've given you some basic recipes to try and personalize. A Mason jar is great for storing salad dressings.

Research shows that women who have a little healthy fat (like olive oil) with their salads are better able to absorb the nutrients!

SALAD IN A JAR

Think of making your salad in layers. Start with a quart-size wide-mouth Mason jar. Begin layering, and before you know it, *voilà*, a perfect salad! Place the dressing at the bottom and pack greens closer to the top to prevent wilting. When you are ready to eat, shake the salad into a bowl and toss gently. Salads may be kept in the refrigerator for a few days before combining, so make a few ahead to save time!

Mason Jars Are Not for Jelly

I like to make double batches of soups, stews, and chilis and freeze planned-overs in pint-size Mason jars, especially in the cooler months. Once the soup is cool, you can put it in a wide-mouth Mason jar. Fill it two-thirds to three-quarters full, leaving room at the top for expansion. If you have a regular jar with a "shoulder" (where the jar curves to the opening), fill it to the shoulder to avoid breakage. Twist the lid on loosely until the meal is completely frozen, and leave a little space between jars in your freezer. You can even slip your jars into clean socks before you put them into the freezer to keep them from hitting one another and breaking. When you remove the jar from the freezer, defrost it with the lid off in the refrigerator rather than on a kitchen countertop to prevent breakage.

10-Layer Salad in a Jar

Makes 1 serving

1st Layer: Salad Dressing

2 to 4 tablespoons of any of the following:
- White Balsamic Vinaigrette (p. 286)
- Fruit Vinaigrette (p. 286)
- Terrific Tahini Dressing (p. 287)
- Avocado-Lime Ranch Dressing (p. 287)

2nd Layer: Crunchy Veggies

Unlimited amounts of the following:
- Asparagus
- Bell peppers
- Broccoli
- Brussels sprouts
- Cabbage
- Celery
- Cucumbers
- Fennel
- Radish
- Red onion
- Shallots
- Snap peas
- String beans

3rd Layer: Protein (optional)

If you decide to skip this layer, use a protein salad such as tuna or chicken salad or bean dip as the 10th layer.

½ cup of any of the following:
- Leftover dinner protein
- Black beans
- Cannellini
- Chickpeas
- Hard-boiled eggs
- Kidney beans
- Lentils

4th Layer: Gluten-Free Grain and/or Roasted or Raw Starchy Veggie (optional)

¼ to ⅓ cup total of any of the following:
- Beets
- Brown rice
- Carrots
- Corn
- Millet
- Quinoa
- Sweet potato
- Winter squash
- Wild rice

5th Layer: Soft Veggies

If you are making your salad ahead of time, add this layer in last before you transport.

Unlimited amounts of the following:
- Artichoke hearts
- Avocado
- Hearts of palm
- Mushrooms
- Olives
- Tomatoes
- Summer squash
- Zucchini

6th Layer: Fresh Fruit (optional)

¼ cup of any of the following:
- Apples (toss first in a little freshly squeezed lemon juice to prevent browning)
- Berries
- Melons
- Pears (toss first in a little freshly squeezed lemon juice to prevent browning)
- Stone fruits

7th Layer: Nuts, Seeds, and Dried Fruit (optional)

Up to ¼ cup of the following:
- Unsweetened coconut
- Nuts
- Seeds

Or 1 tablespoon (maximum) dried fruit

8th Layer: Greens and Sprouts

Unlimited amounts of any of the following:
- Arugula
- Belgian endive
- Butter lettuce
- Curly endive
- Dandelion greens
- Kale
- Mesclun
- Mizuna
- Mustard greens
- Radicchio
- Red leaf lettuce
- Romaine
- Spinach
- Watercress

9th Layer: Fresh herbs

Unlimited amounts of any of the following:
- Broccoli sprouts
- Chives
- Cilantro
- Dill
- Green onions
- Mint
- Oregano
- Parsley
- Pea shoots
- Radish sprouts
- Rosemary

10th Layer: Bean Dip or Prepared Salads

Use a 10th layer only if you are omitting the 3rd layer.

⅓ to ½ cup of any of the following:
- Hummus (p. 292)
- Rosemary White Bean Dip (p. 292)
- Curried Egg Salad (p. 252)
- Orange Chicken Salad (p. 253)

Place the salad dressing (layer 1) in the bottom of a quart-size wide-mouth Mason jar. Proceed to pack the layers above in the order given. Seal the jar and store in the refrigerator. To serve, pour the contents of the jar into a bowl and toss to coat the salad ingredients with dressing.

Asian Chicken Noodle Salad in a Jar

Makes 1 serving

4 tablespoons Cilantro-Peanut Sauce (p. 289)
¼ cup diced cucumber
¼ cup bell pepper matchsticks
¼ cup sliced celery
½ cup cooked organic chicken, shredded
¼ cup shredded carrots
1 cup zucchini noodles (I use raw spiralized zucchini)
2 tablespoons unsalted peanuts, chopped
⅓ cup finely shredded baby kale or spinach
2 tablespoons sliced green onions
2 tablespoons chopped fresh cilantro

Layer all of the ingredients in a quart-size Mason jar in the order given. When ready to serve, dump the contents of the jar into a bowl and toss to coat veggies, chicken, and zucchini noodles with the sauce.

Mango–Black Bean Salad in a Jar

Makes 1 serving

3 tablespoons White Balsamic Vinaigrette (p. 286)
2 tablespoons diced red onion
¼ cup chopped red bell pepper
¼ cup red cabbage, shredded
½ cup cooked black beans
¼ cup corn
½ avocado, peeled, pitted, chopped, and tossed in lime juice
¼ cup peeled, pitted, and chopped mango
3 tablespoons pepitas
2 cups chopped romaine lettuce
2 tablespoons sliced green onions
2 tablespoons chopped fresh cilantro

Layer all of the ingredients in a quart-size Mason jar in the order given. When ready to serve, dump the contents of the jar into a bowl and toss to coat vegetables, fruit, beans, and grain with the vinaigrette.

LUNCH WRAPS

Sometimes you're just in the mood for a sandwich. In this case, create a gluten-free lunch wrap using the concept of salad layering.

Layered Lunch Wrap

Makes 1 serving

Layer your wrap the same way you would layer your salad. Remember, the wrap counts as the "grain" layer. Add crunchy veggies, protein, soft veggies, fruit, nuts or seeds, greens, and herbs, in that order (see the options listed in the recipe for 10-Layer Salad in a Jar, p. 248). Roll it up or fold it burrito-style. Alternatively, you can also use one piece of gluten-free bread as the base and create an open-face sandwich.

PROTEIN SALADS

Protein salads make great snacks. Stuff them in cherry tomatoes or serve them alongside some celery sticks and Mary's Gone Crackers. Experiment with different herbs and spices to add variety.

Curried Egg Salad

Makes 1 serving

    2 large organic, free-range eggs, hard-boiled and chopped
    2 tablespoons olive-oil mayonnaise
    2 tablespoons thinly sliced green onions
    2 tablespoons finely chopped celery

1 teaspoon apple cider vinegar
½ teaspoon Dijon mustard
¼ teaspoon curry powder
¼ teaspoon ground cumin
Sea salt and freshly ground black pepper to taste

Combine all ingredients in a bowl and mix. Season with salt and pepper. Serve on a salad or in a wrap.

Orange Chicken Salad

Makes 1 serving

1 tablespoon orange juice
1 tablespoon white-wine vinegar
1 tablespoon extra-virgin olive oil
¼ teaspoon Everyday Seasoning (p. 284)
½ cup cooked organic chicken, shredded
3 orange sections, peeled and coarsely chopped
3 tablespoons sliced celery
2 tablespoons toasted chopped walnuts
1 tablespoon sliced green onions

To make the dressing, in a small bowl whisk together the orange juice, vinegar, olive oil, and seasoning salt. In another bowl, combine the chicken, orange sections, celery, walnuts, and green onions. Toss the chicken mixture with the dressing and serve on salad or in a wrap.

Dinner

It can be quick and easy to plan a scrumptious and healthy PCOS-friendly dinner. You've seen how I like to "layer" breakfasts and lunch salads. You can use the same approach to make many simple dinners. Layering flavors on your proteins or vegetables can transform a dish. You will never feel deprived or hear, "Chicken again?"

SOUPS, CHILIS, AND STEWS

Soups, chilis, and stews are staples in the Healing PCOS Plan. They are a wonderful way to use up leftover protein and vegetables and keep kitchen cleanup to a minimum, since everything is in one pot. Plus, leftovers make a wonderfully nutritious lunch the next day. Soups, chilis, and stews taste best and are most nutrient rich when you use bone broths. It is very simple to make your own.

Homemade Chicken Bone Broth

Makes 4 quarts

This bone broth is a staple in many of my recipes. It also makes a protein-rich and gut-healing snack. I typically roast an organic chicken every week in the fall and winter and use it to make a batch or two of chicken bone broth to use in my soups and stews.

> Bones from a roasted organic chicken
> 4 quarts water
> Handful of fresh parsley
> 1 onion, coarsely chopped
> 1 carrot, coarsely chopped
> 1 parsnip, coarsely chopped
> 2 celery stalks, coarsely chopped
> 1 whole garlic bulb, halved crosswise
> 1 tablespoon whole peppercorns
> 2 bay leaves
> 1 tablespoon sea salt
> 2 teaspoons apple cider vinegar

Add all of the ingredients to a large stockpot. Bring to a boil and reduce to a simmer. Simmer for 3 hours, skimming foam and excess fat occasionally. (Or place all of the ingredients in a slow cooker and cook on low overnight.) Skim the top, cool, and strain through a sieve into a bowl. Cover and chill about 8 hours. Skim the fat from the surface. Refrigerate the broth in an airtight container for up to five days or freeze it for up to three months.

Variation: To make Homemade Beef Bone Broth, roast 4 pounds of organic beef bones, preferably a mix of marrow bones and bones with a little meat on them, such as oxtail, short ribs, or knuckle bones (cut in half by a butcher), for 40 minutes at 450°F, turning once after 20 minutes, until deeply browned. Place the roasted beef bones and other ingredients in the stockpot and simmer 8 to 24 hours. Cool, strain, and refrigerate as above.

Bone Broth Benefits

Chicken soup will heal more than your soul. This powerhouse contains calcium, magnesium, phosphorus, silicon, sulfur chondroitin, glucosamine, and other trace minerals. Grandma was right, research indicates this ancient home remedy can help with:

Gut health. Bone broth heals, protects, and aids in digestion.

Bones and joints. Glucosamine and chondroitin are the building blocks of healthy cartilage.

Protein. Bone broth is a good source of protein too.

Don't limit your broth just to soups. Spread its benefits by substituting it for water when preparing dishes like rice or vegetables.

Rich and Creamy Chicken Stew

Makes 4 servings

This stew is serious comfort food.

2 quarts organic low-sodium chicken broth or Homemade
    Chicken Bone Broth (p. 254), *divided*
1 cup cooked brown rice
2 teaspoons extra-virgin olive oil
1 small onion, chopped
¼ cup finely chopped shallots
2 cloves garlic, minced
2 cups cooked organic chicken, shredded
2 stalks celery, diced
2 carrots, chopped
1 small zucchini, chopped
1 cup kale, ribs removed, roughly chopped
¼ cup peas
2 bay leaves
1 teaspoon dried thyme
1 teaspoon dried rosemary
1 teaspoon paprika
½ teaspoon cayenne pepper (optional)
¼ cup chopped fresh parsley
Sea salt and black pepper to taste

In a blender, combine 1 quart of chicken broth and the cooked rice and blend until smooth. Set aside. In a large pot, heat the oil and cook the onion, shallots, and garlic until translucent. Add the rice-broth blend, remaining broth, chicken, celery, carrots, zucchini, kale, peas, bay leaves, thyme, rosemary, paprika, and cayenne (if using). Simmer for 45 minutes. Remove the bay leaves and stir in the fresh parsley. Season to taste with salt and pepper.

White Chicken Chili

Makes 6 servings

This is one of my most requested recipes and my go-to for potlucks. This version is on the mild side, so if you like your chili spicy and more flavorful, adjust seasonings to taste before serving.

> 1 tablespoon extra-virgin olive oil
> 1 cup finely chopped onion
> 1 yellow bell pepper, chopped
> 2 small summer squash, chopped
> ⅓ cup chopped celery
> 3 cloves garlic, minced
> 1 tablespoon ground cumin
> ½ teaspoon dried oregano
> 1 teaspoon chili powder
> 2 teaspoons ground coriander
> 1 (4.5-ounce) can chopped green chilies, undrained
> 1 quart organic low-sodium chicken broth or
>   Homemade Chicken Bone Broth (p. 254)
> Juice from ½ lime
> 2 (15.5-ounce) cans cannellini beans, rinsed and drained
>   (mash 1 can of beans with a fork or potato masher)
> 4 cups cooked, shredded organic chicken breast
> Sea salt and freshly ground black pepper to taste
> ¼ cup chopped fresh cilantro
> Sliced jalapeños, salsa, guacamole, sliced green onions,
>   lime wedges (garnish)

Heat the oil in a large heavy pan or Dutch oven over medium heat. Add the onions, bell pepper, summer squash, celery, and garlic and sauté until soft. Add the cumin, oregano, chili powder, and coriander and sauté 1 more minute. Stir in the chilies, chicken broth, and lime juice. Add the beans and chicken. Simmer for 30 minutes. Stir in the cilantro and simmer for 5 more minutes. Serve the chili in individual bowls garnished with jalapeños, salsa, guacamole, green onions, and lime wedges.

Meatball Fagioli

Makes 4 to 6 servings

1 pound grass-fed ground beef, organic ground turkey,
   or organic ground chicken
1 organic, free-range egg, beaten
¼ cup gluten-free bread crumbs
3 tablespoons minced fresh parsley
2 cloves garlic, minced
1 teaspoon Everyday Seasoning (p. 284)
¼ teaspoon dried oregano
2 tablespoons extra-virgin olive oil, *divided*
1 cup chopped onion
1 cup chopped celery
1 cup chopped carrots
3 cloves garlic, minced
1½ quarts organic low-sodium beef broth or
   homemade beef bone broth
1 (15.5-ounce) can red kidney beans, drained and rinsed
1 (15-ounce) can tomato sauce
1 (15-ounce) can fire-roasted tomatoes
2 tablespoons Basil Pesto (p. 289)
3 tablespoons chopped fresh parsley
2 cups shredded cabbage
Freshly ground black pepper to taste

Mix the ground meat, egg, bread crumbs, parsley, garlic, Everyday Seasoning, and oregano in a large bowl. Form into small bite-size meatballs and set aside.

In a large, heavy pot or Dutch oven over medium heat, heat 1 tablespoon of olive oil. Cook one-half of the meatballs until brown on all sides and remove. Cook the remaining meatballs and remove. Add the remaining oil and sauté the onion, celery, and carrots for 4 minutes or until they begin to soften. Add the garlic and sauté for 1 more minute.

Add the beef broth, stir, and scrape up any brown bits from the bottom of the pan. Add the kidney beans, tomato sauce, tomatoes, pesto, and parsley. Simmer for 15 minutes. Add the cabbage and meatballs and simmer for 8 to 10 minutes. Season with black pepper.

Variation: You can make a quick and easy fagioli by skipping the meatball step. Just use browned ground meat, leave out the rest of the meatball ingredients, and continue with the recipe as above.

Spiced Pumpkin Beef Stew

Makes 4 to 6 servings

Be sure to use a tender sugar pumpkin for this recipe. You can also substitute other winter squash like butternut or buttercup.

   1½ pounds grass-fed sirloin, cut into 1-inch cubes (If you cook the stew in a
      slow cooker, you can use a cheaper cut.)
   ½ teaspoon sea salt, plus more to taste
   ¼ teaspoon freshly ground black pepper, plus more to taste
   1 tablespoon extra-virgin olive oil
   1 large onion, chopped
   2 celery ribs, chopped
   2 shallots, minced
   3 cloves garlic, minced
   2 bay leaves
   2 sprigs fresh thyme or ½ teaspoon dried thyme
   1½ teaspoons Pumpkin Pie Spice (p. 285)
   1 tablespoon tomato paste
   1 quart organic low-sodium beef broth or homemade beef bone broth
   2 cups sugar pumpkin, peeled and cubed
   1 bunch kale, ribs removed, roughly chopped
   2 cups cauliflower florets
   1 cup frozen pearl onions
   ⅓ cup chopped fresh parsley (garnish)

Season the beef with ½ teaspoon salt and ¼ teaspoon pepper. Heat the olive oil in a large, heavy pot or Dutch oven over medium heat. Add the beef and brown it on all sides. Remove the beef to a plate and set aside.

Pour off most of the fat from the pot and add the onion, celery, and shallots. Sauté until they are just soft, about 5 minutes. Add the garlic and stir for 1 minute. Add the bay leaves, thyme, Pumpkin Pie Spice, tomato paste, and broth. Scrape up any brown bits from the bottom of the pan. Add the beef, pumpkin, and kale and simmer for 1 hour. Add the cauliflower and pearl onions and cook until the cauliflower is soft, about 20 minutes. Remove the thyme sprig (if using) and bay leaves and adjust the seasoning to taste. Ladle into bowls and garnish with parsley.

White Bean Soup with Basil Pesto

Makes 8 servings

As a PCOS Diva, I avoid cream-based soups, but that doesn't mean I don't yearn for a rich and creamy soup. This soup satisfies that craving. It is made from dried navy beans. I find that the texture of the soup is creamier when I start with dried beans rather than canned, but *you must soak the dried beans overnight in cold water before using them in this recipe.* Make certain that the beans are very soft before blending. You may want to invest in an immersion blender, one of my favorite kitchen tools.

1 pound dried navy beans
3 slices nitrate-free applewood-smoked bacon
1 onion, diced
2 shallots, diced
1 celery rib, diced
2 cloves garlic, sliced
2 quarts organic low-sodium chicken broth or Homemade Chicken Bone Broth
   (p. 254; more if needed to reach desired consistency)
1 bay leaf
Sea salt and freshly ground black pepper to taste
2 cups baby spinach
1 tablespoon freshly squeezed lemon juice
½ cup Basil Pesto (p. 289; garnish)

Place the dried beans in a large bowl, cover them with water, and let them soak overnight. Drain and set aside.

In a large, heavy pot or Dutch oven, cook the bacon until crisp. Remove the bacon from the pot and set aside. To the drippings in the pot, add the onion, shallots, and celery. Cook until soft, 3 to 4 minutes. Add the garlic and stir for 1 minute. If there is any visibly remaining bacon grease, remove it from the pot. Crumble the bacon into the pot. Add the drained beans, broth, and bay leaf. Bring to a boil, reduce the heat, and simmer until the beans are very tender, about 1½ to 2 hours, adding more broth as needed.

Remove the bay leaf. Remove ½ cup of beans for garnish. Use a blender (in batches) or an immersion blender to blend the soup until smooth. Season with salt and pepper. Add the spinach and stir to wilt. Add the lemon juice.

To serve, ladle the soup into eight bowls and garnish each bowl with 1 tablespoon of the reserved beans and 1 tablespoon of pesto.

Lentil Soup

Makes 4 to 6 servings

Lentil Soup is a cinch to make. Lentils cook quickly and are incredibly tasty and inexpensive. I like to put a portion of the soup in the blender to give it a heartier consistency.

2 tablespoons extra-virgin olive oil

2 cups chopped onion

1 cup chopped celery

1 cup chopped carrots

2 cloves garlic, chopped

1 quart organic low-sodium chicken broth or Homemade Chicken Bone Broth (p. 254; more may be needed to thin to desired consistency)

1 bay leaf

1¼ cups dried lentils, rinsed and drained

1 (14.5-ounce) can diced tomatoes in juice, undrained

1 cup kale, ribs removed, roughly chopped

1 cup baby spinach

1 teaspoon ground cumin

½ teaspoon paprika

Sea salt and freshly ground black pepper to taste

1 teaspoon apple cider vinegar (optional)

Chopped fresh cilantro (garnish)

Heat the oil in a large, heavy pot or Dutch oven over medium heat. Add the onions, celery, carrots, and garlic and sauté until vegetables begin to brown, about 15 minutes. Add the chicken broth, bay leaf, lentils, and tomatoes and bring to a boil. Reduce the heat to medium-low, cover, and simmer until the lentils are tender, about 35 minutes. Remove the bay leaf. Transfer 2 cups of the soup (mostly solids) to a blender and puree until smooth. Return the puree to the pot. Thin the soup with more broth by ¼ cupfuls until the desired consistency is reached. Add the kale and spinach and cook until wilted. Season with cumin, paprika, salt, pepper, and vinegar (if using). Garnish with cilantro.

Spring Greens Soup

Makes 6 to 8 servings

You will feel amazing after eating this soup. It tastes even better the next day.

1 tablespoon extra-virgin olive oil

1 tablespoon grass-fed butter

2 large onions, chopped

2 leeks, cleaned and chopped

½ cup dry white wine

1½ quarts organic low-sodium chicken or vegetable broth or Homemade
    Chicken Bone Broth (p. 254)

1 bunch swiss chard or kale (about 1 pound), ribs removed,
    coarsely chopped

1 pound baby spinach

½ cup cooked brown rice

⅓ cup chopped fresh cilantro or parsley

Sea salt and freshly ground black pepper to taste

1 tablespoon freshly squeezed lemon juice, or more to taste

¼ teaspoon cayenne pepper (optional)

Extra-virgin olive oil (garnish)

Heat the oil and butter in a large skillet over medium heat. Add the onions and leeks and cook, stirring frequently, until the onions begin to brown, about 5 minutes. Reduce the heat to low, add the wine, and simmer, stirring occasionally, always covering the pan again, until the onions and leeks are reduced and caramelized, about 25 to 30 minutes.

Pour the broth into a stockpot and bring it to a boil. Reduce the heat to a simmer and add the chard or kale, spinach, onion and leek mixture, and cooked rice. Let the greens wilt, but don't simmer them so long that they lose color; you want them to be a bright green. Add the cilantro or parsley, salt and pepper to taste, lemon juice, and cayenne (if using).

Puree the soup in the pot with an immersion blender until perfectly smooth or use a regular blender in batches (returning them to the pot). Taste, and add more lemon juice or seasonings if desired. Garnish each bowl of soup with a drizzle of olive oil.

SKILLET DINNERS

Mushroom and Leek Chicken Skillet

Makes 4 servings

Bacon makes everything better. Just a few slices give this dish a rich smoky flavor.

> 1 tablespoon extra-virgin olive oil
> 1¼ pounds boneless, skinless organic chicken breasts
> ⅓ cup gluten-free flour
> ½ teaspoon sea salt
> ¼ teaspoon freshly ground black pepper
> 2 slices nitrate-free applewood-smoked bacon
> 8 ounces mushrooms, sliced
> 3 leeks, cleaned well and thinly sliced
> 1 shallot, minced
> 2 cloves garlic, minced
> ½ cup dry white wine
> 1 cup organic low-sodium chicken broth or Homemade Chicken Bone
>   Broth (p. 254)
> Chopped fresh parsley (garnish)

Heat the oil in a large skillet over medium heat. Dredge the chicken breasts in flour and season with sea salt and pepper. Add the chicken to the skillet and sauté for 8 to 10 minutes on each side until cooked through. Remove from the pan and set aside. Add the bacon to the skillet and cook until crispy. Remove the bacon and set aside on a paper towel–lined plate.

Add the mushrooms, leeks, shallot, and garlic to the pan drippings in the skillet and cook until the mushrooms and leeks are soft. Add the white wine and scrape up any brown bits at the bottom of the pan. Add the chicken broth and bring to a simmer. Reduce until the sauce is thickened, about 20 minutes. Add the chicken and crumbled bacon to the skillet. Heat through and serve with pan veggies. Garnish with parsley.

Savory Salisbury Steak

Makes 4 servings

When you are in the mood for a meat and potatoes–style dinner, pair this skillet dinner with Root Veggie Mash and half a plate of nonstarchy vegetables.

1 pound grass-fed ground beef

¼ cup minced fresh parsley

3 green onions, chopped

1 teaspoon sea salt

½ teaspoon freshly ground black pepper

1 tablespoon extra-virgin olive oil

2 cups thinly sliced onions

1 teaspoon honey

2 cloves garlic, minced

1 tablespoon tomato paste

2 cups organic low-sodium beef broth or homemade beef bone broth

¼ cup dry red wine

½ teaspoon dried thyme

3½ teaspoons arrowroot mixed with a little water to make a slurry

Chopped parsley (garnish)

In a large bowl, combine the ground beef, parsley, green onions, salt, and pepper. Divide the mixture evenly and form into four 1-inch-thick oval patties. Heat the oil in a large skillet over medium-high heat. Sauté the patties for 3 to 4 minutes per side until browned. Remove from the pan. Reduce the heat to medium-low and add the onions and honey. Sauté the onions until they are soft and browned, about 20 minutes. Stir in the garlic and tomato paste and cook for 1 minute. Stir in the broth, wine, and thyme. Return the patties to the skillet and the bring sauce to a boil. Reduce the heat to low and add the arrowroot slurry. Simmer for 10 minutes. If the sauce is too thin, add a little more arrowroot and water until the desired consistency is reached. Garnish with parsley.

Shrimp Scampi

Makes 4 servings

Serve this scampi over a cup of blanched spiralized zucchini noodles or roasted spaghetti squash.

2 tablespoons extra-virgin olive oil

1 pound jumbo wild-caught shrimp, peeled and deveined

4 cloves garlic, minced

2 shallots, minced

½ cup dry white wine

Juice of 1 lemon

2 cups kale or spinach, ribs removed, shredded

3 tablespoons grass-fed butter

¼ cup chopped fresh parsley

Zest of 1 lemon
Sea salt and freshly ground black pepper to taste
1 cup chopped and seeded fresh tomatoes (garnish)

Heat a skillet over medium-high heat. Add the olive oil and shrimp and sauté just until the shrimp are cooked through. Remove them to a plate. Add the garlic and shallots to the skillet and sauté until both are fragrant, about 1 minute. Add the white wine, lemon juice, and kale or spinach and raise the heat to high. Let the liquid reduce and the greens wilt for 2 minutes. Whisk in the butter and return the shrimp to the pan. Mix in the parsley and zest and season with salt and pepper. Garnish with chopped tomatoes.

Kitchen Skillet

Makes 4 servings

The Kitchen Skillet is a wonderful way to use any protein or veggies that are left over in your refrigerator at the end of the week. It can be made with previously cooked or uncooked ingredients, and it is completely flexible. Get creative! The key to the Kitchen Skillet is caramelized onion. Cooking the onion is time-consuming, but is well worth it for the extra flavor and sweetness that it adds to any vegetables or protein.

1 tablespoon grass-fed butter
1 large onion, sliced
2 tablespoons extra-virgin olive oil, *divided*
4 cloves garlic, sliced
3 to 4 cups uncooked (or cooked) nonstarchy vegetables,
    cut into bite-size portions
3 to 4 cups cooked lean organic protein, cut into bite-size portions
1 to 2 cups cooked gluten-free grain and/or cooked starchy or root veggie
¼ cup organic low-sodium chicken, beef, or vegetable broth
    or Homemade Chicken Bone Broth (p. 254)
Fresh herbs to taste
Crushed red pepper flakes to taste
Additional seasonings (optional)
Everyday Seasoning (p. 284), Jerk Seasoning (p. 284),
    or Southwest Seasoning (p. 285) to taste
Sea salt and ground black pepper to taste

Heat the butter in a large skillet over medium-low heat. Add the onions and stir occasionally for 30 to 40 minutes until caramelized. Remove the onions from the skillet and set aside.

Reduce the heat to low and add 1 tablespoon of olive oil to the skillet. Add the garlic and sauté, stirring occasionally and taking care not to burn, until golden brown, about 5 minutes. Remove the garlic and set aside.

Raise the heat to medium and add the remaining olive oil to the skillet. Add the raw nonstarchy vegetables and any harder herbs, like rosemary, that require a little more cooking time. Sauté the veggies until they are cooked as desired. (If you are using *cooked* nonstarchy veggies that you would like to use up, skip this cooking step and just add them along with the cooked protein, grains, or starchy vegetables in the next step.)

Add the cooked protein, grains, or starchy vegetables, broth, herbs, crushed red pepper flakes, and additional seasonings (if using) to the skillet and mix well. Stir in the reserved garlic and caramelized onions and heat through. Season with an additional seasoning blend or sea salt and ground black pepper to taste.

TACOS AND FAJITAS

Simplify meal planning by having weekly themes. For example, at my house we do Taco Tuesday. It is quick and easy and shortcuts the meal-planning process—it makes one less day I have to come up with something new and original. It is a comfortable routine that has become a tradition.

5-Layer Tacos

Makes 4 servings

1st Layer: Base

1 to 2 per serving of any of the following:
- Hard corn tortillas
- Soft corn tortillas
- Gluten-free wraps

Unlimited:
- Bibb or romaine lettuce wraps
- Salad greens

2nd Layer: Protein

½ cup per serving of any of the following cooked proteins:
- Beans, refried or whole

- Grass-fed beef, ground or bite-size steak pieces
- Organic chicken, ground or bite-size breast pieces
- Wild-caught fish: haddock, cod, or other wild mild white fish
- Wild-caught shrimp
- Organic ground turkey

Skip the Tilapia

I recommend fish as part of a healthy diet. Not only are fish such as salmon, cod, and haddock loaded with protein, they contain lots of omega-3 essential fatty acids (EFAs), which soothe inflammation, improve insulin sensitivity, and reduce cholesterol. Fish also typically contain omega-6 EFAs, which are inflammatory, but our bodies need them in about a 2 to 1 or 4 to 1 omega-3 to omega-6 ratio. Most tilapia found in grocery stores are farm-raised on a diet of corn and soy and have very low levels of beneficial omega-3 fatty acids and very high levels of omega-6 fatty acids.

3rd Layer: Roasted, Grilled, or Sautéed Veggies

Unlimited of any of the following:
- Asparagus
- Bell peppers
- Onions
- Poblano peppers
- Portobello mushrooms
- Summer squash
- Zucchini

4th Layer: Grains (optional)

⅓ cup per serving of brown rice or quinoa

5th Layer: Toppings

Any or all of the following per serving:
- ½ cup Orange Fennel Slaw (p. 283)
- 2 tablespoons Cashew-Lime Crema (p. 290)
- 2 tablespoons Avocado-Lime Ranch Dressing (p. 287)
- ½ cup Fruit Salsa (p. 291)
- 1 ounce nut-based cheese shreds
- Shredded cabbage

- **Chopped fresh cilantro**
- **Freshly squeezed lime juice**
- **Guacamole**
- **Tomato salsa**
- **Raw veggies such as diced bell pepper, tomato, green onion, red onion, avocado, or jalapeño**

Choose your base. Tacos don't have to be on crunchy corn tortillas. I like to mix it up. I will typically use a grain-based wrap for one taco and a bed of lettuce or a lettuce wrap for my second.

To your base, add the 2nd layer, which can be either freshly cooked or leftover cooked protein. To cook a batch, sauté 1 pound of protein, drain if needed, add ¼ cup water and 2 tablespoons of seasoning (Southwest Seasoning, p. 285, is particularly good here), and cook until well-seasoned throughout; adjust to taste. You can also use Citrus Fajitas (p. 268) for this layer.

For the 3rd layer, toss your veggies in avocado oil and 1 teaspoon of Southwest Seasoning (p. 285) or Everyday Seasoning (p. 284) or marinate in Citrus Fajitas marinade (p. 268) and add to the tacos.

Add the 4th layer only if you are *not* using corn or gluten-free tortillas as your base. To your tacos on lettuce wraps or salad greens, feel free to add brown rice or quinoa.

Finally, crown your glorious creation with toppings!

Veggie Tacos

Makes 4 servings

A spicy and savory meatless meal.

    1 zucchini, cut into ½-inch pieces
    1 yellow summer squash, cut into ½-inch pieces
    1 green bell pepper, cut into ½-inch pieces
    1 red bell pepper, cut into ½-inch pieces
    1 onion, cut into ½-inch pieces
    2 tablespoons extra-virgin olive oil
    2 to 3 tablespoons Southwest Seasoning (p. 285)
    8 organic hard taco shells
    1 (15.5-ounce) can black beans, rinsed and drained
    1 (16-ounce) can refried beans
    ½ cup salsa
    1 avocado, pitted, peeled, and chopped

Preheat the oven to 450°F. In a large bowl, toss the zucchini, squash, peppers, and onions with the olive oil and seasoning. Spread the seasoned vegetables on a rimmed baking sheet and roast for 20 minutes or until soft. Heat the shells for a few minutes in the oven and remove. To plate, divide the warm shells among four plates and fill with the vegetables, black beans, and refried beans. Top with salsa and avocado.

Fish Tacos

Makes 4 servings

I always look for fish tacos on the menu when dining out, as they can often be made gluten free. But I also love making these simple tacos at home.

    8 organic soft corn tortillas
    ⅓ cup gluten-free flour
    1 tablespoon Southwest Seasoning (p. 285)
    Pinch of smoked paprika
    1 to 1½ pounds wild-caught haddock, halibut, snapper, or cod
    2 tablespoons avocado oil
    1 medium red onion, sliced
    Cashew-Lime Crema (p. 290)
    Fruit Salsa made with pineapple (p. 291)

Preheat the oven to 350°F. Wrap the tortillas in foil and heat in the oven until warm.

Combine the flour, Southwest Seasoning, and smoked paprika in a shallow dish. Pat the fish dry, then dredge it in the flour mixture. Heat the avocado oil in a cast-iron skillet over medium-high heat. Add the onion and stir occasionally until soft. Add the fish to pan and cook 2 to 3 minutes per side, turning once, until both sides are browned and the fish is flaky. Remove from the pan.

To plate, divide the warm tortillas among four plates, top with the fish and onion mixture, and then add crema and salsa.

Citrus Fajitas

Makes 4 servings

Use steak (I like flank steak for this), chicken, or shrimp in this recipe. Smoked paprika gives these fajitas a nice flavor.

Marinade

    ⅓ cup freshly squeezed lime juice
    ¼ cup freshly squeezed orange juice

¼ cup unsweetened pineapple juice

2 tablespoons Worcestershire sauce

⅓ cup extra-virgin olive oil

3 cloves garlic, minced

2 teaspoons Southwest Seasoning (p. 285)

1 teaspoon smoked paprika

1 teaspoon sea salt

½ teaspoon freshly ground black pepper

¼ cup chopped fresh cilantro

½ jalapeño pepper, seeded and minced (optional)

Fajitas

1¼ pounds grass-fed steak, organic chicken breast,
   or shelled and deveined wild-caught shrimp

2 tablespoons avocado oil, *divided*

1 large onion, sliced

1 small red bell pepper, sliced

1 small green bell pepper sliced

8 tortillas, gluten-free wraps, lettuce wraps, or salad greens

Combine all of the marinade ingredients in a large shallow baking dish. Place the protein in the marinade and turn it over occasionally during the marinating time. Chicken and steak need to marinate for at least 4 hours, preferably overnight, in the refrigerator. Shrimp only need to marinate for 30 minutes in the refrigerator. (Any longer, and the acid in the marinade will start to break down the delicate shrimp meat and make it mushy.)

Remove the protein from the marinade. Heat a cast-iron grill pan over medium-high heat. Add 1 tablespoon of avocado oil, cook the protein until done, and remove it to a cutting board. Slice chicken and steak across the grain into thin slices.

Add the remaining oil to the grill pan and add the onions and bell peppers. Cook until they are softened and have some browned spots, 5 to 6 minutes, stirring occasionally.

Divide the meat evenly among four plates on a bed of salad greens and top with veggies. Alternatively, divide the meat evenly among 8 tortillas, wraps, or lettuce wraps and top with veggies.

OVEN DINNERS

Garlic Roasted Chicken

Makes 4 to 6 servings

In the fall and winter, I often roast a chicken for Monday's dinner. Roast chicken is delicious, and if you add some root veggies like parsnips, carrots, and sweet potatoes to the pan and serve with a salad, you have a complete PCOS Diva Plate meal. You may prepare and season chicken in advance and refrigerate prior to cooking. I use planned-overs for protein in other dinners, soups, and lunch salads and wraps. Of course, I use the bones to make Homemade Chicken Bone Broth (p. 254). Try this recipe with other seasoning blends too.

    1 5-pound whole organic chicken
    2 lemons, zested and quartered
    1 tablespoon Everyday Seasoning (p. 284)
    4 cloves garlic, minced
    2 tablespoons grass-fed butter, melted
    2 tablespoons extra-virgin olive oil
    5 cloves garlic, crushed
    1 medium onion, halved

Preheat the oven to 400°F. Clean the chicken and pat it dry. Place it in a roasting pan. In a small bowl, combine the lemon zest, Everyday Seasoning, minced garlic, butter, and oil. Spread the mixture on top of the chicken, between the skin and the flesh, and in the cavity. Fill the cavity with the quartered lemons, crushed garlic, and onion. Roast the chicken in the oven for 90 minutes or until the juices run clear and the internal temperature reaches 160°F in the meatiest portion of the chicken, the thigh or under the breast where the thigh meets the breast. Let the chicken cool on the countertop for 15 minutes before carving.

Sesame-Crusted Chicken Strips

Makes 4 servings

My upgraded, but still kid-friendly, version of chicken nuggets. Serve with Spicy Raspberry Dipping Sauce (p. 290).

    2 organic, free-range egg whites
    1 cup sesame seeds

1¼ pounds organic boneless, skinless chicken breast, cut into strips
Sea salt and black pepper to taste
Coconut-oil cooking spray

Preheat the oven to 400°F. Line a rimmed baking sheet with parchment paper. In a small bowl, whisk the egg whites until foamy. In a shallow baking dish, spread the sesame seeds. Dip each chicken strip in the egg white and roll in the sesame seeds. Season the chicken pieces with salt and pepper, place on the prepared baking sheet, and coat lightly with coconut-oil spray. Bake for 10 minutes. Turn the chicken strips over, coat lightly with coconut-oil spray, and bake for 5 to 10 minutes more or until the chicken is cooked through and the interior temperature reaches 160°F.

Lemon-Pepper Chicken Drumsticks

Makes 4 servings

Use this marinade for grilled meats too!

Marinade

4 large cloves garlic, crushed
1 teaspoon Everyday Seasoning (p. 284)
1 teaspoon freshly ground pepper
1 teaspoon dried thyme
2 tablespoons sliced green onions
Zest of 1 lemon
¼ cup freshly squeezed lemon juice
2 tablespoons extra-virgin olive oil
2 tablespoons coconut aminos

Chicken

2 pounds organic skin-on chicken drumsticks

In a large bowl, combine all of the marinade ingredients and mix well. Place the drumsticks in a 9 × 13-inch glass baking dish and pour the marinade over them. Marinate the meat in the refrigerator for at least 2 hours or overnight. Remove the drumsticks from the marinade and grill, or bake on a broiling pan in the oven at 400°F, for 35 to 40 minutes, until the chicken is cooked through and the interior temperature reaches 160°F.

Maple-Mustard Salmon

Makes 4 servings

If you are not sure whether you like salmon, please try this recipe. It will make you a fan. Alternatively, this salmon can be grilled.

Avocado-oil cooking spray
4 (6-ounce) wild-caught salmon fillets, skin on
3 tablespoons maple syrup
1 tablespoon Dijon mustard
1 tablespoon tamari soy sauce or coconut aminos
Juice of ½ lemon
1 clove garlic, minced
⅛ teaspoon sea salt
⅛ teaspoon freshly ground black pepper
1 tablespoon finely sliced green onions (garnish)

Preheat the oven to 400°F. Grease a 9 × 13 × 2-inch baking pan with the cooking spray. Place the salmon in the prepared baking pan, skin side down. In a small bowl, combine the syrup, mustard, soy sauce, lemon juice, and garlic and stir until well blended. Sprinkle the fillets with salt and pepper and then spoon the maple and mustard mixture over the fillets. Bake for 8 to 12 minutes, until the sauce begins to caramelize and the fish flakes easily with a fork. Garnish with green onions.

Horseradish-Encrusted Halibut

Makes 4 servings

Part of my heritage is eastern European, so horseradish was a staple in my grandparents' house. I love using this medicinal root in my meals. It is very stimulating to the body's immune system and is anti-inflammatory. Paired with oily fish, horseradish stimulates digestion. You can substitute salmon or any white firm-fleshed, wild-caught fish in this recipe.

4 (6-ounce) wild-caught halibut fillets
¼ cup olive-oil mayonnaise
1 shallot, finely minced
2 teaspoons Dijon mustard
1 tablespoon prepared horseradish
2 teaspoons freshly squeezed lemon juice
1 teaspoon lemon zest
¼ cup gluten-free bread crumbs

2 tablespoons grass-fed butter, melted
1 tablespoon chopped chives or green onions
1 tablespoon chopped fresh parsley
¼ teaspoon sea salt
¼ teaspoon freshly ground black pepper

Preheat the oven to 400°F. Place the halibut fillets in a 9 × 13 × 2-inch baking pan. In a small bowl, combine the mayonnaise, shallot, mustard, horseradish, lemon juice, and lemon zest. Spread the mayonnaise mixture on top of the fillets in a thin layer. In a small bowl, combine the bread crumbs (to make your own gluten-free bread crumbs, toast gluten-free bread well, let it cool, and then pulse in a blender or food processor), melted butter, chives, parsley, salt, and pepper. Spread the bread-crumb mixture evenly over the halibut fillets. Cover the baking dish with foil and bake for 7 minutes. Remove the foil and bake for 4 minutes more, or until the crumbs are golden brown and the fish flakes easily.

GRILL DINNERS

I love summertime because the cooking is easy. It takes no time to sprinkle a piece of meat, poultry, or fish with a seasoning blend, marinate it in one of my dressings, grill it, and then top it with one of my salsas or sauces. Pair the meat with some grilled veggies and a side salad, and dinner is served. Experiment with lots of different flavor combinations, and you'll never be bored. Your taste buds (and body) will thank you.

Grilled kabobs are easy to make and offer up a complete dinner, if you combine them with a side of my Quinoa Pilaf (p. 279). Flavor the protein by marinating it in a dressing, rubbing it with a seasoning salt, or brushing it with a sauce. I like to combine veggies and even fruit with the meat on my kabobs. The variations are endless, so use your creativity. Below are a couple of my family's favorites.

Chicken and Peach Kabobs

Makes 4 servings

Fruit Vinaigrette (p. 286)
12 wooden skewers, soaked in water

1¼ pounds organic boneless, skinless chicken breasts, cut into 1½-inch pieces

4 fresh small peaches, rinsed and sliced into large cubes, skin on

2 small zucchini, cut into ½-inch rounds

1 red bell pepper, cut into bite-size pieces

1 medium sweet Vidalia onion, cut into bite-size pieces

1 (8-ounce) carton button or baby bella mushrooms, halved

4 cloves garlic, crushed

Avocado oil, for the grill

Make 1 batch of Fruit Vinaigrette (p. 286) using peaches.

Prepare the kabobs by randomly threading the chicken, peaches, zucchini, red bell pepper, onion, and mushrooms onto the soaked wooden skewers. Lay them in a 9 × 13 × 2-inch glass baking pan and drizzle evenly with the vinaigrette. Add the garlic to the pan. Refrigerate the meat for at least 4 hours, up to overnight, turning occasionally to thoroughly coat the kabobs with the marinade.

Use a folded paper towel lightly soaked with avocado oil to coat the cold grill grate. Heat the grill to medium-high. Remove the kabobs from the marinade and grill them, turning every minute or two, until the chicken is thoroughly cooked and no longer pink inside and the interior temperature is 160°F, about 10 minutes.

Caribbean Salmon and Pineapple Kabobs

Makes 4 servings

Marinade

¼ cup freshly squeezed orange juice

¼ cup freshly squeezed lime juice

¼ cup extra-virgin olive oil

¼ cup tamari soy sauce or coconut aminos

1 tablespoon Jerk Seasoning (p. 284)

3 cloves garlic, crushed

¼ cup sliced green onions

1 (2-inch) piece fresh ginger, peeled and sliced

Kabobs

1 pound center-cut wild-caught salmon fillet, skinned, cut into 1-inch cubes

12 wooden skewers, soaked in water

2 cups fresh pineapple, cut into 1-inch cubes

2 small summer squash, cut into ½-inch rounds

1 green bell pepper, cut into bite-size pieces

1 medium sweet Vidalia onion, cut into bite-size pieces
Avocado oil, for the grill

In a medium bowl, combine all the marinade ingredients. Add the cubes of salmon and coat them completely with the marinade. Cover and chill for 1 to 2 hours. Prepare the kabobs by randomly threading the marinated salmon, pineapple, summer squash, pepper, and onion onto the soaked wooden skewers.

Use a folded paper towel lightly soaked with avocado oil to coat the cold grill grate. Heat the grill to medium-high. Grill the kabobs, turning every minute or two, until the salmon is cooked through and opaque, about 10 minutes.

Sides

6-Step Roasted Veggies

Makes 4 servings

Many of my clients who had always used corn as their go-to vegetable side dish (though it's really a starch) have fallen in love with roasted vegetables as an easy-to-make and delicious alternative. Roasting makes the veggies brown and crisp on the outside and caramelizes their natural sugars, making them slightly sweet.

When it comes to roasting veggies, be creative! You can roast veggies you may not have thought about roasting before, like radishes, cabbage, green beans, and sugar snap peas.

Step 1. Preheat the oven to 425°F.

Step 2. Prepare 1 to 2 pounds of vegetables by washing, drying, peeling, and cutting vegetables into uniform-size pieces so they cook evenly.

Step 3. In a large bowl, combine vegetables, aromatics, oil, fresh fruit, and seasonings and toss to coat.

Aromatics: Up to ½ cup onion, leek, shallots, up to 2 tablespoons garlic or ginger.

Oil: 1 to 2 tablespoons of high-heat oil such as avocado or coconut oil.

Fresh fruit: Up to ½ cup chopped pears, chopped apples, cranberries, or grapes.

Seasoning: 1 to 2 teaspoons combination of sea salt, ground black pepper, and spices or Everyday Seasoning (p. 284), Jerk Seasoning (p. 284), or Southwest Seasoning (p. 285).

Step 4. Spread the vegetable mixture out on a rimmed baking sheet. Be sure not to overcrowd the veggies, or you'll end up steaming instead of roasting them.

Step 5. Roast on the middle rack of the oven, tossing the vegetables every 10 to 15 minutes, until they are tender and browned. Most vegetables take 10 to 30 minutes. Root vegetables and winter squashes take 30 to 60 minutes. If you are roasting a variety of vegetables together, you may need to roast in stages. Give the harder, longer-cooking vegetables a head start and then add softer, faster-cooking ones, so they all finish cooking at the same time.

Step 6. Layer on more flavor by adding additional ingredients after roasting:

Fresh greens: Toss with a handful of arugula or baby spinach.

Citrus: Sprinkle with orange, lemon, or lime zest or a squeeze of juice.

Bacon: Sprinkle with 2 to 3 slices crumbled crisp-cooked bacon (everything tastes better with bacon!).

Fresh herbs: Toss with a couple tablespoons of any chopped fresh herbs.

Sauces/dressings: Toss to taste with tamari soy sauce, Tabasco, Sriracha, sambal oelek, Chimichurri Sauce (p. 288), Basil Pesto (p. 289), or Cilantro-Peanut Sauce (p. 289).

Vinegar: Drizzle with 1 to 2 teaspoons of any vinegar to brighten flavors.

Toasted nuts and/or seeds: Add 2 to 3 tablespoons for texture and crunch.

Maple syrup or honey: Drizzle with 1 to 2 teaspoons.

--- In a Pinch ---

For a super quick and easy dinner, roast onions, peppers, a few baby red potatoes, zucchini, and summer squash (remember to use the PCOS Diva Plate ratio here). When they are finished, toss them with cooked and browned Italian chicken sausage and fresh basil and parsley. This dinner works equally as well on the grill (just grill the potatoes in a foil packet).

Roasted Roots

Makes 4 servings

If you've never had a turnips, beets, parsnips, or rutabagas before, you'll be surprised at how tasty they are when roasted.

> 2 pounds root vegetables (a mix of any or all of the following: sweet potatoes, carrots, parsnips, turnips, rutabagas, beets), peeled and cut into 1-inch pieces
> 1 onion, peeled and cut into ⅓-inch wedges
> 2 tablespoons avocado oil
> Sea salt and freshly ground black pepper to taste

Preheat the oven to 425°F. Place the root veggies and onion in a roasting pan (you can also use a rimmed cookie sheet or a 9 × 13-inch pan). Drizzle them with the oil, season with salt and pepper, and toss to coat. Spread the veggies out in the pan, so they are not crowded. Roast for 45 to 50 minutes, tossing every 10 minutes, until they are lightly browned and soft.

Orange Roasted Brussels Sprouts

Makes 4 servings

I never liked brussels sprouts until I learned how to roast them. Brussels sprouts lend themselves well to flavor layering. Bacon, balsamic vinegar, and maple syrup are all delicious on top!

> 1½ pounds brussels sprouts, trimmed and cut in half
> 2 tablespoons avocado oil, *divided*
> Sea salt to taste
> Juice and zest of 1 orange
> 2 teaspoons honey

Preheat the oven to 425°F. In a large bowl, toss the brussels sprouts with 1 tablespoon of oil and a sprinkle of sea salt. Place the sprouts on a rimmed baking sheet in single layer. Roast until the sprouts are tender and caramelized, about 25 to 30 minutes. In a small bowl, whisk together the remaining oil, orange juice, zest, and honey. Toss the cooked brussels sprouts with the orange mixture and serve.

Garlicky Greens

Makes 4 servings

If you've never had sautéed swiss chard, kale, or beet greens, you are missing out! Even the most finicky greens eaters love this recipe.

- 2 tablespoons grass-fed butter
- 1 tablespoon extra-virgin olive oil
- 4 cloves garlic, crushed
- 1 bunch of greens such as red Russian kale, Lacinato kale, mustard greens, spinach, beet greens, or swiss chard, ribs removed, chopped, or bok choy, chopped
- 2 teaspoons tamari soy sauce or coconut aminos
- 1 teaspoon freshly squeezed lemon juice
- 1 to 2 tablespoons sesame seeds (optional)

Melt the butter in a skillet over low heat. Add the garlic and sauté for 1 minute. Add the olive oil and soften the garlic for about 10 minutes, stirring frequently to ensure it doesn't burn. Remove the garlic from the skillet. Keep the garlic-flavored oil/butter in the pan. Increase the heat to medium, place the greens in the skillet, and cover. Cook the greens for 5 to 7 minutes, stirring occasionally until wilted. Remove the greens from the heat, stir in the soy sauce and lemon juice, add the garlic back in if desired, and sprinkle with sesame seeds (if using).

Whipped Butternut Squash

Makes 4 servings

You can use other varieties of squash like buttercup, delicata, or acorn as well.

- 1 small or ½ large butternut squash
- 3 tablespoons grass-fed butter
- 2 teaspoons maple syrup
- ½ teaspoon pure vanilla extract
- ¼ teaspoon freshly grated nutmeg
- Sea salt and freshly ground black pepper to taste

Preheat the oven to 350°F. Cut the squash in half lengthwise and scoop out the seeds. Place the squash halves, cut side down, in a baking dish with enough water to cover the bottom (about ½ inch). Poke a few holes in the skin of the squash with a fork. Cover and bake for 1 hour or until the squash is fork-tender. Scoop the flesh from the skin into a bowl and mash with a potato masher or whip with an immersion blender or handheld mixer while adding in the butter, maple syrup, vanilla, and nutmeg. Season with salt and pepper to taste.

Root Veggie Mash

Makes 4 servings

The mild onion flavor of the leeks makes a nice addition to this mashed root-veggie side dish.

   2 tablespoons grass-fed butter, *divided*
   2 leeks, cleaned and cut into 1-inch pieces
   2 large parsnips, peeled and cut into 1-inch pieces
   2 small unpeeled Yukon Gold potatoes, cut into 1-inch pieces
   2 cups organic low-sodium chicken or vegetable broth or
      Homemade Chicken Bone Broth (p. 254)
   ⅛ teaspoon freshly grated nutmeg
   Sea salt and freshly ground black pepper to taste
   1 tablespoon finely chopped parsley (garnish)

Melt 1 tablespoon of butter in a medium-size saucepan over medium heat. Add the leeks and cook, stirring occasionally, until slightly softened, 5 to 7 minutes. Add the parsnips, potatoes, broth, and nutmeg and bring to a boil, uncovered, stirring occasionally. Reduce the heat and simmer until the vegetables are very tender and most of the liquid is absorbed, about 30 minutes. Remove from the heat, add the remaining butter, and mash with a potato masher (veggies can be a bit chunky). Season with salt and pepper and garnish with parsley.

Quinoa Pilaf

Makes 4 servings

You could use a variety of vegetable and herb combinations in this pilaf. Here is one of my favorites. Be sure to rinse quinoa well before you cook it.

   1 tablespoon extra-virgin olive oil
   2 shallots, chopped
   1 clove garlic, minced
   1 teaspoon Everyday Seasoning (p. 284)
   1 cup dried quinoa

¼ cup dry white wine

1¾ cups organic low-sodium chicken or vegetable broth
     or Homemade Chicken Bone Broth (p. 254)

1 cup baby spinach, chopped

½ cup toasted chopped walnuts

¼ cup chopped fresh parsley

1 medium cucumber, peeled, seeded, and diced into ½-inch pieces

Zest of 1 lemon

Sea salt and freshly ground black pepper to taste

Heat the oil in a large saucepan over medium-high heat. Add the shallots and cook until soft, about 2 minutes. Add the garlic and Everyday Seasoning and stir for 1 minute. Add the quinoa, wine, and broth. Cover the pan, bring to a simmer, and cook until all the liquid has been absorbed and the quinoa is soft, about 15 minutes. Remove from the heat and add the spinach, walnuts, parsley, cucumber, and lemon zest and toss well. Season to taste with sea salt and ground black pepper.

4-Step Grilled Veggies

Makes 4 servings

If you are not a fan of cooked veggies, try grilling them. Like roasting, grilling caramelizes vegetables' natural sugars and the smoky taste from the grill adds another layer of flavor. Plus, grilling is easy, and there is minimal kitchen cleanup. You can enjoy these veggies hot or cold on salads. Use leftovers in soups, frittatas, or on a lunch wrap. Don't be afraid to try veggies that you wouldn't think of for grilling, like romaine lettuce, bok choy, brussels sprouts, leeks, and cauliflower.

Step 1. Cut 1 to 2 pounds of veggies so they are about ¼ to ½ inch thick. It is easy to overcook vegetables cut into smaller pieces, making them soggy.

Step 2. Toss the vegetables in 1 to 2 tablespoons of avocado oil, the ideal oil for grilling because of its high smoke point, and sprinkle with sea salt, ground black pepper, and 1 to 2 teaspoons of Everyday Seasoning (p. 284), Jerk Seasoning (p. 284), or Southwest Seasoning (p. 285). Alternatively, marinate the veggies for 30 minutes in White Balsamic Vinaigrette (p. 286) or the Citrus Fajitas marinade (p. 268).

Step 3. Use a folded paper towel lightly soaked with avocado oil to coat the cold grill grate. Heat the grill to medium-high and grill veggies until grill marks appear. Turn the heat down and cook the vegetables until just before they've reached the desired doneness (they will continue to cook after you take them off the heat) or place them over indirect heat. You don't want the outside to cook too quickly and the inside to be raw.

Grill smaller-cut veggies on skewers or use a grill basket to keep them from falling through the grate. Alternatively, you can cook your veggies in a foil packet. This works well for denser root veggies. Use a 24-inch piece of foil coated with coconut-oil spray. Arrange seasoned and thinly sliced veggies in a single layer, slightly overlapping, leaving a 2-inch border on the sides. Fold the foil over and roll the edges to seal. Place the packet on the grill and cover. Cook until the veggies are tender.

Step 4. Bump up the flavor (optional). Toss the grilled veggies in a dressing or sauce and fresh herbs after they come off the grill.

Grilled Cauliflower Steaks with Sweet Vidalia Onions

Makes 4 servings

Cauliflower is a versatile, low-carb side dish. Serve it roasted, riced, or in steaks. I serve these steaks with Chimichurri Sauce (p. 288) on the side.

- 1 head cauliflower
- 1 large sweet Vidalia onion, sliced into ½-inch rounds
- 3 tablespoons avocado oil, plus more for the grill
- Sea salt and freshly ground black pepper to taste

Remove the leaves and trim the stem of the cauliflower, but do not remove the core. Place the cauliflower core-side down on a cutting board. Slice the cauliflower into four ½-inch "steaks."

Drizzle the cauliflower steaks and onions with avocado oil and season with sea salt and pepper. Use a folded paper towel lightly soaked with avocado oil to coat the cold grill grate. Heat the grill to medium-high. Grill cauliflower steaks and onions until tender and charred in spots, 8 to 10 minutes per side. Oil, season, and grill any loose cauliflower florets in a grill basket, tossing occasionally, until cooked through, 5 to 7 minutes.

Dani's Mediterranean Chopped Salad

Makes 4 servings

One of my favorite side-salad recipes is a very simple but flavorful chopped salad that my friend Dani introduced me to. He grew up on the Mediterranean, and this salad was often on his dinner table when he was growing up. You could also add Kalamata olives, arugula, shredded carrots, and any combination of fresh cilantro, basil, and mint. Sprinkle with toasted pine nuts and add chickpeas for protein to make this a lunch salad.

Juice of 2 lemons
¼ cup extra-virgin olive oil
2 cloves garlic, minced
1 teaspoon sea salt
1 teaspoon freshly ground black pepper
2 cups cherry tomatoes, cut into quarters
1 bell pepper, chopped
3 green onions, thinly sliced
½ medium red onion, diced
2 cups seeded and chopped cucumber
¼ cup chopped fresh parsley

In a pint-size Mason jar, combine lemon juice, olive oil, garlic, sea salt, and black pepper and shake well to blend. In a large bowl, combine the tomatoes, pepper, green onions, red onion, cucumber, and parsley. Pour the lemon-juice dressing on the salad and toss well. Refrigerate for 1 hour before serving to allow the flavors to meld.

Gingered Apple and Apricot Slaw

Makes 4 servings

This slaw tastes equally delicious with chopped firm pear.

⅓ cup plain almond-milk or coconut-milk yogurt
¼ cup olive-oil mayonnaise
2 teaspoons freshly squeezed lemon juice
2 tablespoons white balsamic vinegar
1 teaspoon grated fresh ginger
2 teaspoons poppy seeds
½ teaspoon sea salt
¼ teaspoon freshly ground black pepper
1 small Honeycrisp apple, cut into matchsticks

1 carrot, peeled and shredded
4 cups shredded cabbage
⅓ cup chopped dried apricots
⅓ cup chopped walnuts
2 green onions, thinly sliced
¼ cup pepitas

In a small bowl, whisk together the yogurt, mayonnaise, lemon juice, vinegar, ginger, poppy seeds, salt, and black pepper to make a dressing. In a large bowl, combine the apple, carrot, cabbage, dried apricots, walnuts, green onions, and pepitas and toss with the dressing to coat. Serve chilled.

Orange Fennel Slaw

Makes 4 servings

If you have never had fennel before, I promise you will be pleasantly surprised. It adds wonderful flavor to this salad. If you especially like the anise-like taste, garnish the salad with the chopped fennel fronds.

2 tablespoons freshly squeezed orange juice
2 tablespoons extra-virgin olive oil
1 tablespoon apple cider vinegar
½ teaspoon sea salt
¼ teaspoon freshly ground black pepper
1 carrot, peeled and shredded
2 green onions, sliced
1 large fennel bulb, trimmed and thinly sliced
1 cup shredded red cabbage
2 medium oranges, peeled and cut into small sections
    (add any extra juice from sectioning to dressing)
2 tablespoons dried cranberries

In a pint-size Mason jar, combine the orange juice, olive oil, vinegar, salt, and black pepper and shake well to combine. In a large bowl, combine the carrot, onions, fennel, cabbage, and oranges. Add the dressing and toss well. Top with the cranberries. Serve chilled.

Seasonings, Dressings, and Sauces

SEASONINGS

There are countless varieties of seasoning you can use to flavor protein and veggies. All you have to do is sprinkle it on and grill, roast, or sauté. This is an opportunity to get creative. Develop your signature blend. There are many blends at the grocery store that are tasty too. Just make sure they are free of gluten and MSG and use sea salt. These are my go-to seasonings; they keep one to two years if free from moisture.

Everyday Seasoning

Makes about ⅔ cup

- ¼ cup finely ground sea salt
- 2 tablespoons onion powder
- 2 tablespoons garlic powder
- 1½ tablespoons ground black pepper
- 2 teaspoons celery salt
- 2 teaspoons ground white pepper

Combine all of the ingredients in a pint-size Mason jar and shake well.

Jerk Seasoning

Makes about ¾ cup

- 3 tablespoons finely ground sea salt
- 2 tablespoons ground allspice
- 2 tablespoons dried thyme
- 1 tablespoon coconut sugar
- 2 tablespoons garlic powder
- 1 tablespoon paprika
- 2 teaspoons ground black pepper
- 2 teaspoons ground cinnamon

2 teaspoons freshly grated nutmeg
½ teaspoon cayenne pepper (optional)

Combine all of the ingredients in a pint-size Mason jar and shake well.

Southwest Seasoning

Makes about ½ cup

2 tablespoons chili powder
1 tablespoon ground cumin
1 tablespoon finely ground sea salt
2 teaspoons paprika
2 teaspoons garlic powder
1 teaspoon ground black pepper
1 teaspoon onion powder
1 teaspoon dried oregano
½ teaspoon cayenne pepper (optional)

Combine all of the ingredients in a pint-size Mason jar and shake well.

Pumpkin Pie Spice

Makes about ⅓ cup

¼ cup ground cinnamon
2 teaspoons freshly grated nutmeg
2 teaspoons ground allspice
1 teaspoon ground ginger
½ teaspoon ground cloves

Combine all of the ingredients in a pint-size Mason jar and shake well.

DRESSINGS

The vinaigrette dressings can be drizzled on roasted and grilled veggies as well as poultry and meat and can be used as dipping sauces for snacking on veggies.

I am a huge fan of flavored Modena balsamic vinegars. Although they are pricey, they are also extremely flavorful, and a little goes a long way. I currently have pineapple, peach, lemon, and cranberry-pear white balsamic vinegars as well as strawberry, blueberry, pumpkin spice, and fig red balsamic varieties in my pantry. The salad-dressing combinations are endless!

Flavored extra-virgin olive oils are also delicious. Experiment with different infusions. You can buy them or make them yourself. I love my Meyer lemon– and blood orange–flavored olive oils!

White Balsamic Vinaigrette

Makes about ¾ cup

   ½ cup extra-virgin olive oil
   ¼ cup white balsamic vinegar
   1 teaspoon maple syrup or raw honey
   ½ teaspoon Dijon mustard
   Sea salt and freshly ground black pepper to taste

Combine the oil, vinegar, maple syrup, and mustard in a pint-size Mason jar and shake well. Season with salt and pepper.

Variations: Balsamic vinaigrette can be made with red balsamic vinegar. If using a flavored balsamic vinegar, omit the sweetener. You can also substitute raw apple cider vinegar and play with the mustard. I like to use spicy brown or even whole-grain mustard instead of Dijon.

Fruit Vinaigrette

Makes about ⅔ cup

This recipe is wonderful with fresh fruit in season, like blueberries, peaches, strawberries, or cherries.

¾ cup fresh fruit, coarsely chopped
⅓ cup extra-virgin olive oil
1 to 2 tablespoons white balsamic or apple cider vinegar
Zest and juice of ½ lemon
2 tablespoons chopped shallot
3 fresh basil or mint leaves, chopped
½ teaspoon sea salt
¼ teaspoon freshly ground black pepper

Blend all of the ingredients in a blender or food processor until smooth and creamy. Add a bit of water to thin it to the desired consistency. Adjust the flavors to taste.

Terrific Tahini Dressing

Makes about ⅔ cup

This is a wonderful all-purpose dressing and can be the generous dollop of healthy fat on your PCOS Diva Plate.

¼ cup tahini
3 tablespoons tamari soy sauce or coconut aminos
3 tablespoons extra-virgin olive oil
1 tablespoon toasted sesame oil
1 tablespoon apple cider vinegar
1 clove garlic, minced
1-inch piece fresh ginger, peeled and grated
Juice of ½ lemon
2 teaspoons raw honey (optional)

Blend all of the ingredients in a high-speed blender until smooth, creamy, and emulsified. Add water to thin if desired.

Avocado-Lime Ranch Dressing

Makes about 1 cup

If you miss creamy, dairy-based dressings, then this is the one for you.

1 avocado, pitted and peeled
⅓ cup fresh cilantro
Zest and juice of 1 lime
2 tablespoons extra-virgin olive oil

1 clove garlic, minced
2 green onions, chopped
½ teaspoon sea salt
¼ teaspoon freshly ground black pepper
¼ teaspoon ground cumin
Jalapeño pepper (optional)

Blend all of the ingredients in a high-speed blender until smooth and creamy. Add a bit of water to thin it to the desired consistency. Adjust the flavors to taste.

SAUCES

Stewed Spiced Fruit

Makes about 1 cup

2 teaspoons grass-fed butter
1 cup peeled, chopped fruit
1 date, pitted and chopped
2 teaspoons ground cinnamon, nutmeg, ginger, cloves, or cardamom
   (or a combination)
2 tablespoons water

Heat the butter in a small pan over medium heat. Add the fruit and date and sauté until the fruit begins to soften. Add your chosen spice(s) and water. Cover and cook on low heat, stirring occasionally, until the fruit is soft and tender. Use to top Chia Pudding Parfait (p. 231) or Super-Seed Quick Oats (p. 234). You could also use it like a chutney on protein.

Chimichurri Sauce

Makes about ½ cup

This sauce is delectable on any protein. I especially like it with grilled steak and shrimp. I also like it drizzled over grilled or roasted veggies or even soup. This sauce will only last for a day or two, but you can freeze any remaining sauce in ice-cube trays to drop into soups and stews.

⅓ cup extra-virgin olive oil
⅓ cup fresh basil
⅓ cup fresh cilantro
⅓ cup fresh parsley
1 tablespoon lime juice
1 tablespoon red-wine vinegar
1 clove garlic, minced
½ teaspoon sea salt
¼ teaspoon freshly ground black pepper

Blend all of the ingredients in a high-speed blender until smooth. Adjust the seasonings to taste.

Basil Pesto

Makes about ½ cup

This dairy-free pesto is a perfect addition when drizzled on cooked veggies, protein, salads, or soups, as a spread for your lunch wrap, or tossed with spiralized zucchini noodles.

3 tablespoons pine nuts or chopped raw walnuts
1 cup tightly packed fresh basil
¼ cup extra-virgin olive oil
1 large clove garlic, minced
1 teaspoon freshly squeezed lemon juice
¼ teaspoon sea salt

Lightly toast the nuts in a dry skillet or in the oven. Blend all of the ingredients in a high-speed blender until smooth. Adjust the seasonings to taste.

Cilantro-Peanut Sauce

Makes about 1½ cups

This sauce marries perfectly with the Asian Chicken Noodle Salad in a Jar (p. 251). You can also use it as a dipping sauce for grilled chicken, meat, or shrimp or serve it as a dip for raw vegetables or Fresh Spring Rolls (p. 296) for a snack.

1 cup unsalted smooth or chunky organic peanut butter
½ cup very warm water
½ cup chopped fresh cilantro

⅓ cup tamari soy sauce or coconut aminos
¼ cup tahini
¼ cup rice vinegar
¼ cup green onions, finely chopped
2½ tablespoons grated fresh ginger
2 tablespoons sesame oil
1 tablespoon raw honey
2 cloves garlic, minced
1½ teaspoons Chinese chili paste

Blend all ingredients in a high-speed blender until smooth. Adjust the seasonings to taste. If the sauce is too thick, add a bit more warm water.

Spicy Raspberry Dipping Sauce

Makes about ⅔ cup; 1 serving: 2 tablespoons

I use this sauce for dipping my Sesame-Crusted Chicken Strips (p. 270). You can substitute blueberries or blackberries.

½ cup no-sugar-added raspberry preserves or jam
½ cup frozen raspberries
2 tablespoons white balsamic vinegar
1 teaspoon prepared horseradish (optional)

In a small saucepan over low heat, combine the raspberry preserves, frozen raspberries, and vinegar. Bring to a low simmer and cook until slightly thickened. Stir in the horseradish (if using).

Cashew-Lime Crema

Makes about ½ cup

If you miss sour cream, this is a nice alternative. This also tastes great as a topping for tacos and roasted veggies. It will last in the refrigerator three to four days and can be frozen in ice-cube trays for up to six months.

½ cup raw cashews
¼ cup fresh cilantro
¼ cup filtered water, plus more for soaking
1 clove garlic, minced
1 lime, juiced
½ teaspoon chili powder

½ teaspoon garlic powder
½ teaspoon sea salt
¼ teaspoon freshly ground black pepper

In a large bowl, cover the cashews with boiling water and soak for 1 hour (or soak in room-temperature water for 6 to 8 hours or overnight). Drain and rinse the cashews. Place all of the ingredients in a high-speed blender and blend until smooth, adding more water until the desired consistency is reached. Adjust the seasonings to taste.

Lemon-Dijon Sauce

Makes 4 servings

This sauce can be used on an endless variety of steamed or roasted veggies.

2 teaspoons extra-virgin olive oil
1 teaspoon lemon zest
2 tablespoons freshly squeezed lemon juice
½ teaspoon Dijon mustard
Sea salt and freshly ground black pepper to taste
1 tablespoon finely chopped parsley

Combine oil, zest, juice, and mustard. Whisk to emulsify. Season with salt and pepper and chopped parsley.

Fruit Salsa

Makes about 2 cups; 1 serving: ⅓ cup

Fruit salsa is a wonderful complement to grilled, baked, or roasted protein and is, of course, wonderful for taco combinations. I like to use stone fruits, strawberries, or pineapple.

2 cups chopped fruit
¼ cup finely sliced green onions
¼ cup minced fresh cilantro
1 clove garlic, minced
Zest and juice of 1 lime
Sea salt to taste

In a bowl, combine all of the ingredients. Chill for 30 minutes to allow the flavors to meld before serving.

🌿 Dips

Hummus

Makes about 3 cups

This recipe is from my dear Lebanese friend Mirna and is my favorite take on hummus. She insists you must not use canned chickpeas. Rather, soak dried beans overnight and cook them with ½ teaspoon salt, either in a pressure cooker or on the stovetop, for about an hour until *very* tender.

> 3 cups cooked and drained chickpeas
> ½ cup tahini
> Juice of 2 lemons
> 3 cloves garlic, minced
> ½ cup extra-virgin olive oil
> Sea salt to taste
> Extra-virgin olive oil, ground cumin, chopped parsley,
>   toasted pine nuts (garnish)

Process all of the ingredients in a food processor until smooth and creamy. Thin with a little water until the desired consistency is reached. Adjust the seasoning and lemon juice to taste.

To serve, drizzle with olive oil and garnish with cumin, parsley, and pine nuts. Store in an airtight container in the refrigerator for up to four days.

Rosemary White Bean Dip

Makes about 1½ cups

The taste of Tuscany in a bowl! This appetizer is always requested by my friends when we get together for ladies' night.

> 1½ cups cooked or 2 (15-ounce) cans, rinsed and drained,
>   Great Northern beans or cannellini beans
> 2 cloves garlic, minced
> 1 tablespoon finely chopped fresh rosemary
> 1 green onion, sliced
> ½ teaspoon sea salt
> Zest and juice of ½ lemon
> ¼ cup extra-virgin olive oil

In a food processor or high-speed blender, combine the beans, garlic, rosemary, and green onions. Pulse in the salt and lemon zest and juice. Pulse until the mixture is coarsely pureed, then thin with a little water until the desired consistency is reached. With the food processor or blender running, slowly add the olive oil to emulsify. Once incorporated, scrape the sides of the bowl or blender, and process until the dip is smooth. Adjust the seasoning to taste. Store in an airtight container in the refrigerator for up to four days.

🌿 Snacks and Sweet Treats

Most of us can get from breakfast to lunch without a snack. The time between lunch and dinner is another matter. During this time, we PCOS Divas need a snack to keep our blood sugar even and prevent us from getting too hungry and making desperate choices at dinnertime. Again, preparation is key. *Plan your snacks out in advance.* As you plan your snacks, keep a few things in mind.

Experiment with pairing a carbohydrate with a protein and a fat. Eating carbohydrates by themselves can trigger a blood sugar spike. Later, when your blood sugar falls, it will cause more cravings, fatigue, and moodiness. The carb and protein combination should give you longer-lasting energy without the crash.

Try to focus on savory snacks. Reserve sweets for an occasional, mindfully indulgent sweet treat. This generally includes fruit, which is ideally reserved for breakfast in a smoothie, oatmeal, or chia pudding or as a garnish in a salsa or salad with a meal.

Use the protein bars, muffins, egg muffin cups, and chia pudding from the breakfast recipes as snacks.

Pair bean dips, tapenade, or salad dressings with veggie sticks or seed crackers like Mary's Gone Crackers.

Turn lunch salads, such as tuna, chicken, or egg salad, into snack options.

As always, experiment and see what works best for you.

DAILY SNACKS

Sweet Spiced Pepitas

Makes 2 cups

> 2 cups pepitas
> 2 tablespoons coconut sugar
> 1 tablespoon virgin coconut oil (liquid)
> 2 teaspoons Pumpkin Pie Spice (p. 285)
> ½ teaspoon finely ground sea salt

Preheat the oven to 300°F. Line a cookie sheet with parchment paper. Combine the pepitas, coconut sugar, coconut oil, Pumpkin Pie Spice, and salt in a bowl and mix well. Spread the seeds in a single layer on the prepared cookie sheet. Bake for 20 minutes, stirring occasionally. The seeds will be golden and crunchy when done. Cool and store in an airtight container.

Variation: To make Savory Spiced Pepitas, substitute Southwest Seasoning (p. 285) for Pumpkin Pie Spice, reduce the amount of coconut sugar to 2 teaspoons, and replace the coconut oil with lime juice.

5-Layer Trail Mix

Makes 4½ cups; 1 serving: ⅓ cup

About once a month I make a huge batch of trail mix. It is easy to go overboard, so be sure to portion it out and keep to one serving per day. Store it in an airtight container and consume it within one month, although a batch never lasts that long in my house.

1st Layer: Raw Nuts

> 2 cups of any combination of the following:
> - Almonds
> - Brazil nuts
> - Cashews
> - Hazelnuts
> - Macadamia nuts
> - Pecans
> - Pine nuts
> - Pistachios
> - Walnuts

2nd Layer: Seeds

1 cup of any combination of the following:
- Hemp seeds
- Pepitas
- Sunflower seeds

3rd Layer: Dried Fruit

Choose dried fruit with as little added sugar and as few preservatives as possible. Unsweetened and unsulfured dried fruit is best.

1 cup of any combination of the following:
- Apples, chopped
- Apricots, chopped
- Blueberries
- Cherries
- Cranberries
- Dates, chopped
- Figs, chopped
- Goji berries
- Mango, chopped
- Pineapple, chopped

4th Layer: Sweet Treats

½ cup of any combination of the following:
- Cacao nibs
- Coconut flakes
- Dark chocolate chips
- Dark chocolate–covered nuts or dried fruit

5th Layer: Dash of Spice (optional)

Any of the following ground spices:
- Cardamom
- Cayenne
- Cinnamon
- Nutmeg
- Sea salt

Combine all of the ingredients in a large bowl and mix well. Store in large glass jars.

Avocado-Bacon Deviled Eggs

Makes 6 servings

This twist on deviled eggs makes for a flavorful, filling snack.

- 2 slices nitrate-free applewood-smoked bacon, diced
- 6 large peeled, hard-boiled organic, free-range eggs
- 1 avocado, halved, pitted, and peeled
- 2½ tablespoons olive-oil mayonnaise
- 2 tablespoons chopped fresh cilantro
- 2 tablespoons finely chopped green onions
- 1 tablespoon freshly squeezed lemon juice
- Zest of 1 lemon
- 1 teaspoon Dijon mustard
- Garlic powder to taste
- Sea salt and freshly ground black pepper to taste
- Cayenne pepper (optional)
- Paprika (garnish)

Cook the bacon until crispy. Transfer to a paper towel–lined plate, cool, and crumble. Cut the eggs in half lengthwise, scoop out the yolks, and place them in small a bowl. Add the avocado, mayonnaise, cilantro, green onions, lemon juice, zest, and mustard and mash until combined and creamy. Season to taste with garlic powder, sea salt, black pepper, and cayenne (if using). Pipe the filling into the egg whites with a pastry bag. Sprinkle with bacon bits and garnish with paprika.

Fresh Spring Rolls

Makes 4 servings

These rolls are a bit of work, but certainly worth it. I love to bring these to holiday parties. Cut the rolls in half on the diagonal and place them on a pretty platter with Cilantro-Peanut Sauce (p. 289) on the side.

- 8 (8-inch) rice paper rounds
- 16 large cooked, peeled wild-caught shrimp or
  2 cups shredded cooked chicken
- 1 cup boiling water
- 1 cup shredded carrot
- 1 cup thinly sliced Napa cabbage
- 1 cup bean sprouts
- ½ cup julienne-sliced, peeled, and seeded cucumber

1 avocado, peeled, pitted, and sliced
4 tablespoons chopped fresh cilantro
8 large fresh basil leaves, halved lengthwise

Cut each shrimp in half lengthwise and set aside. Fill a large, shallow baking dish with the water. Place 1 rice-paper round in the water and soak until pliable, about 30 seconds. Carefully transfer the wrapper to a paper towel and turn once to blot dry. On the bottom half of the wrapper, arrange a ⅛ portion of each of the veggies (carrot, cabbage, spouts, cucumber, and avocado) and ½ tablespoon cilantro. Fold the bottom edge of the wrapper toward the center and roll up the wrapper halfway, making sure to wrap tightly around the filling. Tuck 2 basil-leaf halves along the inside crease of the half-rolled wrapper. Arrange 4 pieces of shrimp, cut sides up, or ¼ cup shredded chicken along the crease. Fold the right and left edges of the wrapper over the filling and finish rolling up. Repeat with the remaining wrappers, veggies, cilantro, basil, and shrimp or chicken. Transfer the rolls to a plate and cover with dampened paper towels until serving time. Serve with Cilantro-Peanut Sauce.

Sundried Tomato and Basil-Stuffed Mushrooms

Makes 5 servings

Packed with omega 3–rich walnuts, these stuffed mushrooms are rich and toothsome.

20 large white button stuffing mushrooms
1 tablespoon extra-virgin olive oil
1 small shallot, minced
½ cup diced bell pepper (I use a mix of red and green)
2 cloves garlic, minced
2 green onions, finely chopped
1 cup baby spinach, chopped
¼ cup jarred sundried tomatoes in oil, drained, chopped
¼ cup chopped fresh basil
2 tablespoons chopped fresh parsley
Sea salt and freshly ground black pepper to taste
¾ cup raw walnuts, finely chopped
2 teaspoons red balsamic vinegar

Preheat the oven to 375°F. Place the mushrooms on a rimmed cookie sheet and bake for 10 to 15 minutes, until the mushrooms have softened and released their moisture. Remove the mushrooms from the oven and transfer them to a serving dish. Remove the stems from the mushrooms and set aside. Brush the mushroom caps with olive oil, return them to the cookie sheet, stem side up, and bake for 10 minutes.

While the mushrooms are in the oven, make the filling. Dice the mushroom stems. Heat the olive oil in a sauté pan over medium heat. Add the mushroom stems, shallot, bell pepper, garlic, green onions, spinach, tomatoes, basil, parsley, salt, and pepper. Sauté the veggies until they are tender and spinach is wilted. Add the walnuts and balsamic vinegar and remove from the heat.

Remove the mushrooms from the oven. Pour off any water that has accumulated in the mushrooms. Spoon the filling into the mushrooms and bake for an additional 10 to 12 minutes, until the tops are golden. Serve warm.

Additional Daily Snack Ideas

- ¼ cup Hummus (p. 292) or Rosemary White Bean Dip (p. 292) with veggies
- Scoop of tuna salad, Curried Egg Salad (p. 252), or Orange Chicken Salad (p. 253) in half of an avocado
- 1 cup roasted brussels sprouts or cauliflower with Terrific Tahini Dressing (p. 287)
- 4 celery sticks and 1 tablespoon nut or seed butter with 5 to 6 raisins or dried cranberries
- Raw veggies with a couple tablespoons of dressing, sauce, or guacamole
- ½ avocado mashed and seasoned with lime juice, sea salt, and cayenne on seed crackers
- 4 to 5 small gluten-free meatballs
- 1 serving of nitrate-free jerky
- 1 hard-boiled egg and some veggie sticks
- 2 ounces of leftover meat with dressing, sauce, or guacamole
- 3 cucumber sandwiches (3 small pieces of meat or spoons of lunch salad between 6 crunchy cucumber slices)
- A cold chicken drumstick and some veggies
- 4 large cooked wild-caught shrimp with 1 tablespoon organic cocktail sauce
- 1 cup of soup or broth (Who said soup is just for meals?)

SWEET TREATS

Everyone needs a little sweet treat now and then, whether for a cele-bration or just a well-deserved indulgence. As you indulge, remember that sweet treats are just that—treats. They are not meant for every day. Luckily, PCOS Divas know how to indulge in a treat like this mind-fully. Plan for it, and make something delicious and aligned with the PCOS Diva lifestyle: gluten free, dairy free, processed-soy free, and whole-foods based. There's no sense in indulging if you are just going to feel lousy later! You'll find lots of additional ideas on PCOSDiva .com/sweettreats.

If you don't think you can eat just one serving of these sweet treats, you may be better off purchasing a single-serving dairy-free, gluten-free dessert at your grocery store.

Spiced Berry Dream

Makes 4 servings

Use a cultured coconut-milk or almond-milk yogurt. My favorite brand is Kite Hill. Its vanilla Artisan Almond Milk Yogurt is to die for.

   2 cups vanilla-flavored coconut- or almond-milk yogurt
   ½ teaspoon ground cinnamon
   ¼ teaspoon freshly grated nutmeg
   2 pints fresh blueberries, blackberries, raspberries, or strawberries
      (or a combination)
   ¼ cup sliced almonds, toasted

In a bowl, combine the yogurt, cinnamon, and nutmeg. Divide the berries be-tween four dessert bowls, and top each with ½ cup of the yogurt mixture and 1 tablespoon of toasted sliced almonds.

Buckeyes

Makes 2 dozen balls; 1 serving: 2 balls

This is strictly a special holiday-time treat, but certainly a better choice than fudge. Be sure you only indulge in one or two and share the rest. Warming the honey helps it combine with the other ingredients.

1 cup PCOS Diva Power Protein, vanilla or chocolate
   (or similar protein powder)
½ cup natural crunchy nut butter
½ cup raw honey, warmed
1 teaspoon pure vanilla extract
½ cup bittersweet chocolate chips, at least 60 percent cacao

In a medium bowl, combine the protein powder, nut butter, honey, and vanilla. Blend with an electric mixer until combined. Form the mixture into 1-inch balls, place on a cookie sheet lined with wax or parchment paper, and refrigerate until set. Melt the chocolate in a small heavy saucepan or double boiler. Using a skewer, lift a ball and dip it halfway into the chocolate. Place the ball on a cookie sheet lined with wax or parchment paper and refrigerate until set.

Chocolate Chip Cookies

Makes 24 cookies; 1 serving: 2 cookies

These are sure to satisfy your cookie craving. And the high-fat content of the almond butter and flour will help you to feel satiated after eating one or two cookies—you won't feel the need to eat the whole batch.

⅓ cup finely ground almond flour
⅓ cup coconut sugar
½ teaspoon baking soda
1 cup almond butter (I like Barney Butter brand for these)
1 teaspoon pure vanilla extract
1 organic, free-range egg
½ cup bittersweet chocolate chips (at least 60 percent cacao)

Preheat the oven to 350°F. Line a baking sheet with parchment paper. In a large bowl, combine the almond four, coconut sugar, and baking soda and mix well. Add the nut butter, vanilla, and egg and mix until combined. Gently fold in the chips. Drop the dough onto the cookie sheet by spoonfuls and gently flatten each one to a 1-inch-diameter disk. Bake for 10 minutes, or until golden brown. Cool on a baking rack.

Diva Hot Chocolate

Makes 1 serving

Sometimes a cup of rich hot chocolate soothes my soul. By swapping coconut milk for cow's milk and using a small amount of sweetener, you can enjoy a cup every now and then without guilt.

1 cup unsweetened coconut milk (for a very decadent version, use 1 cup from a
    13.5-ounce can of full-fat coconut milk)
1½ tablespoons cocoa (the higher quality the cocoa, the better your hot
    chocolate will taste) or raw cacao powder (I like Navitas Naturals)
1 tablespoon coconut nectar, raw honey, or coconut sugar
¼ teaspoon pure vanilla extract
¼ teaspoon pure peppermint extract

Combine the milk, cocoa, sweetener, and extracts in a saucepan over medium heat and stir occasionally with a whisk until the mixture is at your desired temperature. (Do not allow your milk to boil!) Pour it into your favorite mug and enjoy!

Pumpkin Pie Crème Brûlée

Makes 6 servings

Crème brûlée is my absolute favorite dessert. My body can no longer tolerate even a few bites of the dairy version, so I had to develop a dairy-free recipe.

4 organic, free-range egg yolks
2 organic, free-range eggs
1 (13.5-ounce) can full-fat coconut milk
⅓ cup coconut sugar, plus 2 tablespoons, *divided*
½ cup organic canned pumpkin
1 tablespoon Pumpkin Pie Spice (p. 285)
1 vanilla bean scraped or 1 tablespoon pure vanilla extract
Coconut-oil cooking spray

Preheat the oven to 300°F. In a high-speed blender, blend the egg yolks, eggs, coconut milk, ⅓ cup coconut sugar, canned pumpkin, Pumpkin Pie Spice, and vanilla bean or extract. Pour the mixture into six ramekins that have been coated with coconut-oil spray. Place the ramekins in a large baking dish and add hot water until it comes halfway up the side of the ramekins. Bake for 40 minutes or until set. Cool and chill until ready to serve. Sprinkle the remaining 2 tablespoons of coconut sugar evenly over the tops of the ramekins. Torch or broil them until crispy and brown.

Variation: To make the classic vanilla-flavored dessert, omit the pumpkin and the Pumpkin Pie Spice.

PCOS Diva Symptom Assessment

Please complete the PCOS Diva Symptom Assessment before you begin the 21-Day Plan and then again when you finish. This exercise will help you to identify your symptoms and measure how much they improve in only 21 days. You will feel so much better after completing the plan that you may forget how lousy you felt at the beginning. Comparing the before and after scores will help you to quantify the change.

On a scale from 1 to 5, rate your current PCOS symptoms.

1 = I do not experience this symptom.

2 = The symptom is a minor problem. I notice the symptom, but it is not a big concern.

3 = The symptom is a moderate problem for me. It impacts my life, but I can manage it.

4 = The symptom is a serious problem. I continually struggle with it.

5 = The symptom is severe. I can barely function.

Date:

SYMPTOM					
Acne	1	2	3	4	5
Bloating	1	2	3	4	5
Irritability	1	2	3	4	5
Fatigue	1	2	3	4	5
Moodiness	1	2	3	4	5
Stress	1	2	3	4	5
Brain Fog	1	2	3	4	5
Low Libido	1	2	3	4	5
Weight Gain	1	2	3	4	5
Irregular Cycle	1	2	3	4	5
Blood-Sugar Swings	1	2	3	4	5
Other _____	1	2	3	4	5

Total of Each Column

Total Score

Knowledge Is Power

FURTHER RESOURCES
FOR PCOS DIVAS

PCOS Nonprofit Associations

PCOS Awareness Association (pcosaa.org)

PCOS Challenge (pcoschallenge.org)

Verity (verity-pcos.org.uk)

Amy's Go-to Experts

You can find many of these experts on the PCOSDiva podcast.

PCOS

Lara Briden, ND (LaraBriden.com)

Poppy Daniels, MD (DrPoppy.com)

Shawna Darou, ND (darouwellness.com)

Nancy Dunne, ND (pcosconsultations.com)

Felice Gersh, MD (felicelgershmd.com)

Dian Ginsberg, MD (womensspecialtyhealthcare.com)

Brooke Kalanic, ND (betterbydrbrooke.com)

Meaghan Kirschling, DC, APRN, RN, MS
(oneagorahealth.com)

Karen Leggett, MD (drkarenleggett.com)

Carol Lourie, ND, LAc (carollourie.com)

Fiona McCulloch, ND (drfionand.com)

Margrit Mikulis, ND (livingnaturalinc.com)

Rebecca Murray, APRN, FNP, CDE
(instituteofhormonalbalance.com)

Katherine Sherif, MD (hospitals.jefferson.edu/departments-and
-services/womens-primary-care.html)

Fertility

Rashmi Kudesia, MD, MSc (houstonivf.net)

Victoria Maizes, MD (victoriamaizesmd.com)

Marc Perloe, MD (arcfertility.com)

Aimee Raupp (aimeeraupp.com)

Aumatma Shah, ND (draumatma.com)

Marc Sklar, DC (MarcSklar.com and Reproductive
Wellness.com)

Thyroid

Shannon Garrett, BS, RN, CNN (holisticthyroidcare.net)

Izabella Wentz, PharmD, FASCP (thyroidpharmacist.com)

Magdalena Wszelaki (hormonesbalance.com)

Anxiety

Megan Buer (harmony-restored.com)

Trudy Scott, CN (everywomanover29.com)

Emotional or Disordered Eating

Stephanie Dodier, CCN (stephaniedodier.com)

Melissa McCreery, PhD, MA (toomuchonherplate.com)

Books on Amy's Shelf

PCOS and Hormones

The Adrenal Reset Diet, by Alan Christianson, NMD

8 Steps to Reverse Your PCOS, by Fiona McCulloch, ND

Hashimoto's Protocol, by Izabella Wentz, PharmD, FASCP

The Hormone Cure, by Sara Gottfried, MD

The Hormone Link, by Margarita Ochoa Maya, MD

Integrative Women's Health, by Victoria Maizes, MD, and
   Tieraona Low Dog, MD

Life Is Your Best Medicine, by Tieraona Low Dog, MD

The Natural Diet Solution for PCOS and Infertility, by Nancy
   Dunne, ND and Bill Slater, M.B.A

A Patient's Guide to PCOS, by Walter Futterweit, MD

PCOS, by Samuel Thatcher, MD

The Period Repair Manual, by Lara Briden, ND

The Ultimate PCOS Handbook, by Colette Harris and
   Theresa Cheung

Think like a PCOS Diva

Beautiful You, by Rosie Molinary

Begin with Yes, by Paul S. Boynton

The Big Leap, by Gay Hendricks

Big Magic, by Elizabeth Gilbert

Bonjour Happiness, by Jamie Cat Callan

A Course in Weight Loss, by Marianne Williamson

The Desire Map, by Danielle LaPorte

The Four Agreements, by Don Miguel Ruiz

The Gift of an Ordinary Day, by Katrina Kenison

Gifts of Imperfection, by Brené Brown

Honor Yourself, by Patricia Spadaro

Nothing Changes Until You Do, by Mike Robbins

A Philosopher's Notes, by Brian Johnson

The Rhythm of Life, by Matthew Kelly

The War of Art, by Steven Pressfield

You Can Heal Your Life, by Louise Hay

Live like a PCOS Diva

The Life-Changing Magic of Tidying Up, by Marie Kondo

The Tapping Solution, by Nick Ortner

The Tapping Solution for Weight Loss and Body Confidence, by
   Jessica Ortner

Find a Doctor

American Association of Naturopathic Physicians
   (naturopathic.org)

The Institute of Functional Medicine (ifm.org)

Acknowledgments

My little girl, Lila, has a 40 percent chance of inheriting my PCOS genes. I'm determined to forge a new path for her, so if she is diagnosed with PCOS, she doesn't feel the fear and negativity I once did. I'd much rather have her experience the diagnosis as an opportunity to live life like a PCOS Diva. Thank you, Lila, for inspiring me and being the sparkly exclamation point to our family. And to my boys, Clayton and Rhett, I am so happy that I was able to reclaim my health and life, so that I could be the best mom to you that I could be. You make me so proud.

To my husband, Cliff, who has always pushed me to step beyond my self-imposed limits. You knew I had a story to tell and a greater purpose. Thank you for encouraging me every step of the way. Without your unending support, wisdom, and expertise, PCOS Diva and this book would not have been possible. I love and appreciate you.

And of course, thank you to the original PCOS Diva—my mom. I owe you so much.

Nancy Foti, PCOS Diva Content Manager, writer, and collaborator extraordinaire, thank you for sharing your incredible talent and your time over the last four years; it has been an adventure. And to the rest of the team, Carrie Dawe, Ariela Torgersen, Silvanna Topete, and Emily Otterman, thank you for your support, encouragement, and care.

To my agent, John Maas, and the team at Sterling Lord Literistic, thank you for believing in my message and helping me refine and share it with the world. I'm so grateful to my publisher, HarperOne, for understanding the importance of this book and being willing to take this first-time author under its wings. Thank you to my talented editor, Julia Pastore, who has championed my message, and to the rest of the team at HarperOne, who have worked hard to turn a dream into reality.

And finally, to my fellow PCOS Divas. I'm honored to share this journey with you. May we all continue to move beyond the struggles of PCOS, to live the lives we were meant to live, without being held back by PCOS. May PCOS be the catalyst for tremendous positive transformation in our lives.

With a heart filled with love and gratitude, *thank you*!

Notes

Chapter 2. Why You Feel Lousy

16 *Polycystic ovary syndrome (PCOS) is one of the most common . . . :* "Infertility FAQs," Centers for Disease Control and Prevention, March 30, 2017, https://www.cdc.gov/reproductivehealth/infertility/index.htm.

16 *As calculated employing the widely used . . . :* Susan Sirmans and Kirsten Pate, "Epidemiology, Diagnosis, and Management of Polycystic Ovary Syndrome," *Clinical Epidemiology* (2013): 1, doi:10.2147/clep.s37559.

16 *PCOS affects approximately 15 to 20 percent of women worldwide . . . :* "PCOS Support Groups," PCOS Foundation, http://pcosfoundation.org/support-groups.

16 *It is present throughout a woman's life . . . :* Samuel S. Thatcher, *PCOS: The Hidden Epidemic* (Indianapolis: Perspectives Press, 2000), 320.

16 *In addition, women with PCOS have . . . :* "Diabetes Home," Centers for Disease Control and Prevention, October 11, 2016, https://www.cdc.gov/diabetes/library/spotlights/pcos.html.

16 *They are also more likely to develop . . . :* "Polycystic Ovary Syndrome," womenshealth.gov, July 26, 2017, https://www.womenshealth.gov/a-z-topics/polycystic-ovary-syndrome.

17 *Polycystic ovaries:* Samuel S. Thatcher, "PCOS 101," http://memberfiles.freewebs.com/26/91/38059126/documents/2005%20HS%20and%20PCOS%20Thatcher%20MD.pdf.

17 *High levels of insulin, insulin resistance:* Stephenson et al., "Luteal Start Vaginal Micronized Progesterone"; Pedro Acién et al., "Insulin, Androgens, and Obesity in Women with and Without Polycystic Ovary Syndrome: A Heterogeneous Group of Disorders," *Fertility and Sterility* 72/1 (July 1999): 32–40, doi:10.1016/s0015-0282(99)00184-3; Nancy Dunne and Bill Slater, *The Natural Diet Solution for PCOS and Infertility: How to Manage Polycystic Ovary Syndrome Naturally* (Seattle: Health Solutions Press, 2005), 28.

17 *Easy weight gain:* Charles J. Glueck et al., "Obesity and Extreme Obesity, Manifest by Ages 20–24 Years, Continuing Through 32–41 Years in Women, Should Alert Physicians to the Diagnostic Likelihood of Polycystic

Ovary Syndrome as a Reversible Underlying Endocrinopathy," *European Journal of Obstetrics & Gynecology and Reproductive Biology* 122/2 (October 1, 2005): 206–12, doi:10.1016/j.ejogrb.2005.03.010; H. J. Teede et al., "Body Mass Index as a Predictor of Polycystic Ovary Syndrome Risk: Results of a Longitudinal Cohort Study," *The Endocrine Society's 92nd Annual Meeting, June 19–22, 2010, San Diego, P2-414*, June 19, 2010, http://dx.doi.org/10.1210/endo-meetings .2010.PART2.P9.P2-414.

17   *obesity:* Walter Futterweit, and George Ryan, *A Patient's Guide to PCOS: Understanding and Reversing Polycystic Ovarian Syndrome* (New York: Holt, 2006), 19.

17   *Fertility issues:* Thatcher, *PCOS*, 12.

17   *Acne:* Futterweit and Ryan, *A Patient's Guide to PCOS*, 17.

17   *Depression:* Amanda A. Deeks, Melanie E. Gibson-Helm, and Helena J. Teede, "Anxiety and Depression in Polycystic Ovary Syndrome: A Comprehensive Investigation," *Fertility and Sterility* 93/7 (February 1, 2010): 2421–23, doi:10.1016/j.fertnstert.2009.09.018; Sudhindra Mohan Bhattacharya and Ayan Jha, "Prevalence and Risk of Depressive Disorders in Women with Polycystic Ovary Syndrome (PCOS)," *Fertility and Sterility* 94/1 (November 6, 2009): 357–59, doi:10.1016/j.fertnstert.2009.09.025; Varvara Laggari et al., "Anxiety and Depression in Adolescents with Polycystic Ovary Syndrome and Mayer-Rokitansky-Küster-Hauser Syndrome," *Journal of Psychosomatic Obstetrics & Gynecology* 30/2 (2009): 83–88, doi:10.1080/01674820802546204.

17   *Anxiety:* Tsilchorozidou, Honour, and Conway, "Altered Cortisol Metabolism in Polycystic Ovary Syndrome"; Shabir et al., "Morning Plasma Cortisol Is Low"; Pasquali and Gambineri, "Cortisol and the Polycystic Ovary Syndrome."

17   *High levels of androgens:* Dominik Rachoń and Helena Teede, "Ovarian Function and Obesity—Interrelationship, Impact on Women's Reproductive Lifespan, and Treatment Options," *Molecular and Cellular Endocrinology* 316/2 (March 25, 2010): 172–79, doi:10.1016/j.mce.2009.09.026; Mitlitsky, "7 Common Symptoms Associated with Low Progesterone."

17   *Irregular menstruation:* Futterweit and Ryan, *A Patient's Guide to PCOS*, 11.

17   *Sleep apnea:* Futterweit and Ryan, *A Patient's Guide to PCOS*, 21.

17   *Gray-white breast discharge:* Futterweit and Ryan, *A Patient's Guide to PCOS*, 20.

17   *Scalp hair loss:* Futterweit and Ryan, *A Patient's Guide to PCOS*, 15.

17   *Darkening skin areas:* Futterweit and Ryan, *A Patient's Guide to PCOS*, 19.

19   *Between 50 and 70 percent of women with PCOS have . . .:* Richard S. Legro, V. Daniel Castracane, and Robert P. Kauffman, "Detecting Insulin Resistance in Polycystic Ovary Syndrome: Purposes and Pitfalls," *Obstetrical & Gynecological Survey* 59/2 (February 1, 2004): 141–54, doi:10.1097/01.ogx .0000109523.25076.e2.

19   *Insulin resistance may be caused . . .:* "Prediabetes and Insulin Resistance,"
National Institute of Diabetes and Digestive and Kidney Diseases, August 1,
2009, https://www.niddk.nih.gov/health-information/diabetes/overview/what
-is-diabetes/prediabetes-insulin-resistance.

19   *Although insulin resistance is often associated with obesity . . .:* Thozhukat,
Sathyapalan and Stephen L. Atkin, "Mediators of Inflammation in Polycystic
Ovary Syndrome in Relation to Adiposity," *Mediators of Inflammation*, March
18, 2010, https://www.hindawi.com/journals/mi/2010/758656/; A. Dunaif
et al., "Profound Peripheral Insulin Resistance, Independent of Obesity,
in Polycystic Ovary Syndrome," *Diabetes* 38/9 (September 1989): 1165–74,
doi:10.2337/diabetes.38.9.1165.

19   *Research also indicates that the birth control pill . . .:* Adeola A. Adeniji
et al., "Metabolic Effects of a Commonly Used Combined Hormonal Oral
Contraceptive in Women with and Without Polycystic Ovary Syndrome,"
Journal of Women's Health 25/6 (January 1, 1970): 638–45, doi:10.1089/jwh
.2015.5418; R. Jeffrey Chang et al., "Insulin Resistance in Nonobese Patients
with Polycystic Ovarian Disease," *Journal of Clinical Endocrinology & Metabolism*
57/2 (August 1983): 356–59, doi:10.1210/jcem-57-2-356.

20   *Researchers disagree about whether hyperinsulinemia . . .:* Richard S.
Legro, "Hyperandrogenism and Hyperinsulinemia," *Global Library of Women's
Medicine*, 2008, doi:10.3843/glowm.10303.

21   *This androgen excess, or hyperandrogenism . . .:* L. Pal, *Polycystic Ovary
Syndrome: Current and Emerging Concepts* (New York: Springer, 2014); Bulent O.
Yildiz et al., "Stability of Adrenocortical Steroidogenesis over Time in Healthy
Women and Women with Polycystic Ovary Syndrome," *Journal of Clinical
Endocrinology & Metabolism* 89/11 (November 2004): 5558–62, doi:10.1210
/jc.2004-0934.

22   *Girls who experience early puberty . . .:* Fionna McCulloch, "PCOS: Treating Adrenal Androgen Excess," *Naturopathic Doctor News and Review*, January 30,
2015, http://ndnr.com/womens-health/pcos-treating-adrenal-androgen-excess/.

22   *Genetics:* Yildiz et al., "Stability of Adrenocortical Steroidogenesis."

22   *Individual hypersensitivity to a normal amount . . .:* Lara Briden, "Causes
of Androgen Excess in Women," *Lara Briden's Healthy Hormone Blog*, May 25,
2017, http://www.larabriden.com/causes-androgen-excess-in-women/.

22   *In fact, research indicates that many women . . .:* Tasoula Tsilchorozidou,
John W. Honour, and Gerard S. Conway, "Altered Cortisol Metabolism in
Polycystic Ovary Syndrome: Insulin Enhances 5α-Reduction but Not the
Elevated Adrenal Steroid Production Rates," *Journal of Clinical Endocrinology
& Metabolism* 88/12 (April 26, 2011): 5907–913, doi:10.1210/jc.2003–030240;
Iram Shabir et al., "Morning Plasma Cortisol Is Low Among Obese Women
with Polycystic Ovary Syndrome," *Gynecological Endocrinology* 29/12 (December
2013): 1045–047, doi:10.3109/09513590.2013.829449; Renato Pasquali and
Alessandra Gambineri, "Cortisol and the Polycystic Ovary Syndrome,"
Medscape, 2012, https://www.medscape.com/viewarticle/773775.

22   *Some doctors recommend supplemental progesterone . . .:* Mary D. Stephenson et al., "Luteal Start Vaginal Micronized Progesterone Improves Pregnancy Success in Women with Recurrent Pregnancy Loss," *Fertility and Sterility* 107/3 (March 2017), doi:10.1016/j.fertnstert.2016.11.029.

23   *Signs of Low Progesterone:* Chris Mitlitsky, "7 Common Symptoms Associated with Low Progesterone," *Dr. Tami,* June 26, 2015, https://www .drtami.com/7-common-symptoms-associated-with-low-progesterone/.

23   *As a result, it can cause changes in vaginal bleeding . . .:* "Progestin (Oral Route, Parenteral Route, Vaginal Route) Side Effects," *Mayo Clinic,* March 1, 2017, http://www.mayoclinic.org/drugs-supplements/progestin-oral-route -parenteral-route-vaginal-route/side-effects/DRG-20069443.

24   *If the thyroid is not functioning properly . . .:* Kris Poppe, Brigitte Velkeniers, and Daniel Glinoer, "Thyroid Disease and Female Reproduction," *Clinical Endocrinology* 66/3 (March 2007): 309–21, doi:10.1111/j.1365-2265 .2007.02752.x.

24   *"Think of PCOS as being in an extended state . . .:* Fiona McCulloch, *8 Steps to Reverse Your PCOS: A Proven Program to Reset Your Hormones, Repair Your Metabolism, and Restore Your Fertility* (Austin, TX: Greenleaf Book Group, 2016), 66–69.

25   *Signs of Thyroid Dysfunction:* "The Difference Between Hypothyroidism and Hyperthyroidism," *Piedmont Healthcare,* accessed October 24, 2017, https://www.piedmont.org/living-better/the-difference-between -hypothyroidism-and-hyperthyroidism.

27   *According to integrative physician Felice Gersh . . .:* Felice Gersh, "PCOS Inflammation: Transform from Inflamed to Tamed," *PCOS Diva,* May 23, 2015, https://pcosdiva.com/2015/05/pcos-and-inflammation-transform -from-inflamed-to-tamed/.

27   *And recent research suggests that women with PCOS . . .:* Héctor F. Escobar-Morreale, Manuel Luque-Ramírez, and Frank González, "Circulating Inflammatory Markers in Polycystic Ovary Syndrome: A Systematic Review and Metaanalysis," *Fertility and Sterility* 95/3 (March 1, 2011), doi:10.1016 /j.fertnstert.2010.11.036.

27   *Although the exact cause of PCOS is unknown . . .:* S. L. Kristensen et al., "A Very Large Proportion of Young Danish Women Have Polycystic Ovaries: Is a Revision of the Rotterdam Criteria Needed?" *Human Reproduction* 25/12 (December 2010): 3117–22, doi:10.1093/humrep/deq273; Richard S. Legro and Jerome F. Strauss, "Molecular Progress in Infertility: Polycystic Ovary Syndrome," *Fertility and Sterility* 78/3 (August 29, 2002): 569–76, doi:10.1016 /s0015-0282(02)03275-2.

27   *With regard to genetics, studies show . . .:* Futterweit and Ryan, *A Patient's Guide to PCOS,* 11.

28   *It is possible that a mother's obesity . . .:* Evanthia Diamanti-Kandarakis, Charikleia Christakou, and Evangelos Marinakis, "Phenotypes and Envi-

ronmental Factors: Their Influence in PCOS," *Current Pharmaceutical Design* 18/3 (2012): 270–82, doi:10.2174/138161212799040457.

28 *Similarly, about 30 percent of women . . . :* Angela Best Boss, Evelina Weidman Sterling, and Jerald S. Goldstein, *Living with PCOS: Polycystic Ovary Syndrome* (Omaha: Addicus Books, 2009), 3.

29 *These were developed by the European Society . . . :* R. Zawadaki and M. Dockerty, "Diagnostic Criteria for Polycystic Ovarian Syndrome: Towards a Rational Approach," in A. Dunaif et al., eds., *Current Issues in Endocrinology and Metabolism: Polycystic Ovarian Syndrome* (Boston: Blackwell Scientific, 1992), 337.

30 *For those taking pills with higher levels . . . :* R. E. Roach et al., "The Risk of Heart Attack and Stroke in Women Using Birth Control Pills," *Cochrane*, August 27, 2015, http://www.cochrane.org/CD011054/FERTILREG _risk-heart-attack-and-stroke-women-using-birth-control-pills.

30 *Studies show that with certain types . . . :* George Mastorakos et al., "Effects of Two Forms of Combined Oral Contraceptives on Carbohydrate Metabolism in Adolescents with Polycystic Ovary Syndrome," *Fertility and Sterility* 85/2 (February 2, 2006): 420–27, doi:10.1016/j.fertnstert.2005.07.1306; Abbey B. Berenson et al., "Effect of Injectable and Oral Contraceptives on Glucose and Insulin Levels," *Obstetrics & Gynecology* 117/1 (January 2011): 41–47, doi:10.1097/aog.0b013e318202ac23; T. Piltonen et al., "Oral, Transdermal and Vaginal Combined Contraceptives Induce an Increase in Markers of Chronic Inflammation and Impair Insulin Sensitivity in Young Healthy Normal-Weight Women: A Randomized Study," *Human Reproduction* 27/10 (July 18, 2012): 3046–56, doi:10.1093/humrep/des225.

30 *Researchers believe that this may have . . . :* I. F. Godsland et al., "Insulin Resistance, Secretion, and Metabolism in Users of Oral Contraceptives," *Journal of Clinical Endocrinology & Metabolism* 74/1 (January 1, 1992): 64–70, doi:10.1210/jc.74.1.64.

31 *Estrogen promotes the growth of yeast . . . :* Gilbert G. Donders, Gert Bellen, and Werner Mendling, "Management of Recurrent Vulvo-Vaginal Candidosis as a Chronic Illness," *Gynecologic and Obstetric Investigation* 70/4 (October 16, 2010): 306–21, doi:10.1159/000314022; G. Cheng, K. M. Yeater, and L. L. Hoyer, "Cellular and Molecular Biology of Candida albicans Estrogen Response," *Eukaryotic Cell* 5/1 (January 01, 2006): 180–91, doi:10.1128/ec .5.1.180-191.2006.

31 *Unfortunately, according to a National Institutes of Health . . . :* "National Institutes of Health Evidence-based Methodology Workshop on Polycystic Ovary Syndrome, Executive Summary," *National Institutes of Health*, December 3, 2012, https://prevention.nih.gov/docs/programs/pcos/FinalReport.pdf.

32 *Metformin is widely acknowledged to deplete . . . :* David S. H. Bell, "Metformin-Induced Vitamin B_{12} Deficiency Presenting as a Peripheral Neuropathy," *Southern Medical Journal* 103/3 (March 2010): 265–67, doi:10.1097 /smj.0b013e3181ce0e4d.

32   *It is not meant to treat insulin resistance . . .:* R. Jeffrey Chang, "Insulin Resistance in Nonobese Patients with Polycystic Ovarian Disease," *Journal of Clinical Endocrinology & Metabolism* 57/2 (August 1, 1983): 356–59, doi:10.1210/jcem-57-2-356; L. Ibanez et al., "Sensitization to Insulin Induces Ovulation in Nonobese Adolescents with Anovulatory Hyperandrogenism," *Journal of Clinical Endocrinology & Metabolism* 86/8 (August 1, 2001): 3595–98, doi:10.1210/jc.86.8.3595.

32   *In women, it has been found . . .:* I. I. Müderris, F. Bayram, and M. Güven, "Treatment of Hirsutism with Lowest-Dose Flutamide (62.5 mg/day)," *Gynecological Endocrinology* 14/1 (2000): 38–41, doi:10.3109/09513590009167658.

32   *and mild to moderate acne:* Enrico Carmina and Rogerio A. Lobo, "A Comparison of the Relative Efficacy of Antiandrogens for the Treatment of Acne in Hyperandrogenic Women," *Clinical Endocrinology* 57/2 (August 2, 2002): 231–34, doi:10.1046/j.1365-2265.2002.01594.x.

32   *Some studies indicate it works . . .:* Leonello Cusan et al., "Comparison of Flutamide and Spironolactone in the Treatment of Hirsutism," *Obstetrical & Gynecological Survey* 49/7 (May 6, 2016): 481–83, doi:10.1097/00006254-199407000-00020.

33   *In fact, many doctors will not prescribe . . .:* "Flutamide (oral)," *University of Michigan Health Services*, December 15, 2010, http://www.uofmhealth.org/node/663457.

33   *Doctors and researchers agree that . . .:* Kathleen M. Hoeger, "Obesity and Lifestyle Management in Polycystic Ovary Syndrome," *Clinical Obstetrics and Gynecology* 50/1 (May 2007): 277–94, doi:10.1097/grf.0b013e31802f54c8; Lisa J. Moran et al., "Effects of Lifestyle Modification in Polycystic Ovarian Syndrome," *Reproductive BioMedicine Online* 12/5 (May 2006): 569–78, doi:10.1016/s1472-6483(10)61182-0; W. C. Knowler et al., "Reduction in the Incidence of Type 2 Diabetes with Lifestyle Intervention or Metformin," *New England Journal of Medicine* 346/6 (February 7, 2002): 393–403, doi:10.1056/nejmoa012512; Thomas Tang et al., "Combined Lifestyle Modification and Metformin in Obese Patients with Polycystic Ovary Syndrome: A Randomized, Placebo-Controlled, Double-Blind Multicentre Study," *Obstetrical & Gynecological Survey* 61/2 (September 31, 2005): 108–9, doi:10.1097/01.ogx.0000197800.07214.dc; Robert Norman et al. [Davies, Lord, Moran], "The Role of Lifestyle Modification in Polycystic Ovary Syndrome," *Trends in Endocrinology and Metabolism* 13/6 (August 1, 2002): 251–57, https://doi.org/10.1016/S1043-2760(02)00612-4; Kathleen M. Hoeger, "Role of Lifestyle Modification in the Management of Polycystic Ovary Syndrome," *Best Practice & Research, Clinical Endocrinology & Metabolism* 20/2 (June 2006): 293–310, doi:10.1016/j.beem.2006.03.008.

33   *Managing diet, lifestyle, and emotional health . . .:* Colette Harris and Theresa Cheung, *The Ultimate PCOS Handbook: Lose Weight, Boost Fertility, Clear Skin and Restore Self-Esteem* (San Francisco: Conari, 2012), 28.

33   *hormonal balance, and help get your insulin . . .:* Lisa J. Moran et al., "Treatment of Obesity in Polycystic Ovary Syndrome: A Position Statement of the Androgen Excess and Polycystic Ovary Syndrome Society," *Fertility and Sterility* 92/6 (2009): 1966–82, doi:10.1016/j.fertnstert.2008.09.018; Robert Ross et al., "Reduction in Obesity and Related Comorbid Conditions After Diet-Induced Weight Loss or Exercise-Induced Weight Loss in Men," *Annals of Internal Medicine* 133/2 (July 18, 2000): 92, doi:10.7326/0003-4819-133-2-200007180-00008; C. L. Harrison et al., "Exercise Therapy in Polycystic Ovary Syndrome: A Systematic Review," *Human Reproduction Update* 17/2 (September 10, 2010): 171–83, doi:10.1093/humupd/dmq045.

33   *Before you know it, your symptoms will . . .:* Thatcher, "PCOS 101."

Chapter 3. Think like a PCOS Diva

46   *Your body's ability to signal . . .:* Kristen L. Knutson, "Impact of Sleep and Sleep Loss on Glucose Homeostasis and Appetite Regulation," *Sleep Medicine Clinics* 2/2 (June 2007): 187–97, doi:10.1016/j.jsmc.2007.03.004; "Sleep and Disease Risk," *Healthy Sleep*, Division of Sleep Medicine at Harvard Medical School, December 18, 2007, http://healthysleep.med.harvard.edu/healthy/matters/consequences/sleep-and-disease-risk.

Chapter 4. Eat like a PCOS Diva

50   *In fact, a startling number of us . . .:* K. F. Michelmore, A. H. Balen, and D. B. Dunger, "Polycystic Ovaries and Eating Disorders: Are They Related?" *Human Reproduction* 16/4 (April 1, 2001): 765–69, doi:10.1093/humrep/16.4.765.

50   *Interpersonal issues, such as . . .:* "Factors That May Contribute to Eating Disorders," *National Eating Disorders Association*, accessed October 25, 2017, https://www.nationaleatingdisorders.org/factors-may-contribute-eating-disorders.

52   *In fact, nutrigenomics . . .:* M. Nathaniel Mead, "Nutrigenomics: The Genome–Food Interface," *Environmental Health Perspectives* 115/12 (December 2007), doi:10.1289/ehp.115-a582.

52   *These interactions may even play . . .:* John M. Berardi, "Nutrigenomics: This Research Changes Everything," *Precision Nutrition*, May 1, 2014, http://www.precisionnutrition.com/nutrigenomics-research.

52   *Studies demonstrate that adding apples . . .:* Jeanelle Boyer and Rui Hai Liu, "Apple Phytochemicals and Their Health Benefits," *Nutrition Journal* 3/1 (May 12, 2004), doi:10.1186/1475-2891-3-5.

52   *Adding an avocado per day to an already . . .:* "Avocados," *The World's Healthiest Foods*, May 23, 2017, http://www.whfoods.com/genpage.php?tname=foodspice&dbid=5.

52   *Berries are packed with immune-boosting . . .:* Tsuyoshi Goto et al., "Tiliroside, a Glycosidic Flavonoid, Ameliorates Obesity-Induced Metabolic Disorders via Activation of Adiponectin Signaling Followed by Enhancement

of Fatty Acid Oxidation in Liver and Skeletal Muscle in Obese–Diabetic Mice," *Journal of Nutritional Biochemistry* 23/7 (July 2012): 768–76, doi:10.1016 /j.jnutbio.2011.04.001; Çetin Çekiç and Mustafa Özgen, "Comparison of Antioxidant Capacity and Phytochemical Properties of Wild and Cultivated Red Raspberries (*Rubus idaeus* L.)," *Journal of Food Composition and Analysis* 23/6 (September 2010): 540–44, doi:10.1016/j.jfca.2009.07.002; Camille S. Bowen-Forbes, Yanjun Zhang, and Muraleedharan G. Nair, "Anthocyanin Content, Antioxidant, Anti-Inflammatory and Anticancer Properties of Blackberry and Raspberry Fruits," *Journal of Food Composition and Analysis* 23/6 (September 2010): 554–60, doi:10.1016/j.jfca.2009.08.012.

52   *Researchers are learning that phytonutrients . . .*: Chie Morimoto et al., "Anti-obese Action of Raspberry Ketone," *Life Sciences* 77/2 (May 2005): 194–204, doi:10.1016/j.lfs.2004.12.029.

53   *Brown rice contains magnesium . . .*: M. Kazemzadeh et al., "Effect of Brown Rice Consumption on Inflammatory Marker and Cardiovascular Risk Factors Among Overweight and Obese Non-menopausal Female Adults," *International Journal of Preventive Medicine* 5/4 (April 2014): 478–88, https:// www.ncbi.nlm.nih.gov/pmc/articles/PMC4018597/.

53   *and manganese for bone and thyroid health . . .*: "Manganese," *University of Maryland Medical Center*, May 31, 2013, http://www.umm.edu/health/medical /altmed/supplement/manganese.

53   *Rich in antioxidants, cinnamon . . .*: Jeff G. Wang et al., "The Effect of Cinnamon Extract on Insulin Resistance Parameters in Polycystic Ovary Syndrome: A Pilot Study," *Fertility and Sterility* 88/1 (July 2007): 240–43, doi:10.1016/j.fertnstert.2006.11.082.

53   *Some studies indicate that it may also . . .*: Daniel H. Kort and Roger A. Lobo, "Preliminary Evidence that Cinnamon Improves Menstrual Cyclicity in Women with Polycystic Ovary Syndrome," *Obstetrical & Gynecological Survey* 70/2 (November 2014): 94–95, doi:10.1097/01.ogx.0000461902.16853.84.

53   *Chocolate containing 70 percent cacao . . .*: David L. Katz, Kim Doughty, and Ather Ali, "Cocoa and Chocolate in Human Health and Disease," *Antioxidants & Redox Signaling* 15/10 (November 15, 2011): 2779–811, doi:10.1089/ars.2010.3697.

53   *It can also improve mood . . .*: Joseph Nordqvist, "Chocolate: Health Benefits, Facts, and Research," *Medical News Today*, June 1, 2016, https:// www.medicalnewstoday.com/articles/270272.php.

53   *As an added bonus, it contains . . .*: Megan Ware, "Magnesium: Health Benefits, Sources, and Risks," *Medical News Today*, September 25, 2017, https:// www.medicalnewstoday.com/articles/286839.php.

53   *Green tea contains a high concentration . . .*: Bhardwaj Pooja and Khanna Deepa, "Green Tea Catechins: Defensive Role in Cardiovascular Disorders," *Chinese Journal of Natural Medicines* 11/4 (July 2013): 345–53, doi:10.3724 /sp.j.1009.2013.00345; Yoshihiro Kokubo et al., "The Impact of Green Tea and Coffee Consumption on the Reduced Risk of Stroke Incidence in

Japanese Population," *Stroke* 44 (March 2013): 1369–74, doi.org/10.1161 /STROKEAHA.111.677500.

53   *Because of its circulatory benefits . . .:* "Health Benefits of Green Tea," *WebMD*, September 13, 2013, https://www.webmd.com/food-recipes/features /health-benefits-of-green-tea#1.

54   *It contains water, protein, fat . . .:* Katherine M. Phillips, Monica H. Carlsen, and Rune Blomhoff, "Total Antioxidant Content of Alternatives to Refined Sugar," *Journal of the American Dietetic Association* 109/1 (January 2009): 64–71, doi:10.1016/j.jada.2008.10.014.

54   *EFAs help regulate hormone function . . .:* Barry Sears and Mary Perry, "The Role of Fatty Acids in Insulin Resistance," *Lipids in Health and Disease* 14/1 (September 29, 2015), doi:10.1186/s12944-015-0123-1.

54   *Thanks to the high fiber content . . .:* Julie-Anne Nazare et al., "Modulation of the Postprandial Phase by β-Glucan in Overweight Subjects: Effects on Glucose and Insulin Kinetics," *Molecular Nutrition & Food Research* 53/3 (March 2009): 361–69, doi:10.1002/mnfr.200800023; A. L. Jenkins et al., "Depression of the Glycemic Index by High Levels of β-Glucan Fiber in Two Functional Foods Tested in Type 2 Diabetes," *European Journal of Clinical Nutrition* 56/7 (July 2002): 622–28, doi:10.1038/sj.ejcn.1601367; N. Tapola et al., "Glycemic Responses of Oat Bran Products in Type 2 Diabetic Patients," *Nutrition, Metabolism and Cardiovascular Diseases* 15/4 (August 2005): 255–61, doi:10.1016/j.numecd.2004.09.003.

58   *In fact, much of the world's adult population . . . :* "NIH Lactose Intolerance Conference-Panel Statement," *National Institutes of Health*, February 24, 2010, https://consensus.nih.gov/2010/lactosestatement.htm.

59   *In addition, your body may struggle to manage . . . :* G. Kristjánsson, P. Venge, and R. Hällgren, "Mucosal Reactivity to Cow's Milk Protein in Coeliac Disease," *Clinical & Experimental Immunology* 147/3 (March 2007): 449–55, doi:10.1111/j.1365-2249.2007.03298.x; Amy Myers, "The Dangers of Dairy," Amy Myers MD, July 18, 2017, https://www.amymyersmd.com/2013 /04/the-dangers-of-dairy/.

59   *Soy is also a goitrogen . . . :* Izabella Wentz, "What Are Goitrogens and Do They Matter with Hashimoto's?" *Dr. Izabella Wentz, Pharm D*, August 07, 2017, https://thyroidpharmacist.com/articles/what-are-goitrogens-and-do -they-matter-with-hashimotos.

59   *Research tells us that intermittent fasting . . . :* Adrienne R. Barnosky et al., "Intermittent Fasting vs. Daily Calorie Restriction for Type 2 Diabetes Prevention: A Review of Human Findings," *Translational Research* 164/4 (October 2014): 302–11, doi:10.1016/j.trsl.2014.05.013.

59   *fight stress and inflammation . . . :* J. B. Johnson et al., "Alternate Day Calorie Restriction Improves Clinical Findings and Reduces Markers of Oxidative Stress and Inflammation in Overweight Adults with Moderate Asthma," *Free Radical Biology and Medicine*, November 1, 2007, doi:10.1016 /j.freeradbiomed.2006.12.005.

59   *reduce depression and improve brain . . .:* Valter D. Longo and Mark P. Mattson, "Fasting: Molecular Mechanisms and Clinical Applications," *Cell Metabolism* 19/2 (January 4, 2016): 181–92, doi:10.1016/j.cmet.2013.12.008; J. Lee, K. B. Seroogy, and M. P. Mattson, "Dietary Restriction Enhances Neurogenesis and Up-regulates Neurotrophin Expression in the Hippocampus of Adult Mice," *Journal of Neurochemistry* 81 (January 21, 2002): 57–59, doi:10.1046/j.1471–4159.81.s1.19_4.x; Jaewon Lee et al., "Dietary Restriction Increases the Number of Newly Generated Neural Cells, and Induces BDNF Expression, in the Dentate Gyrus of Rats," *Journal of Molecular Neuroscience* 15/2 (October 2000): 99–108, doi:10.1385/jmn:15:2:99.

64   *That's about 20 teaspoons . . .:* "How Much Is Too Much?" *Sugar Science, UCSF,* December 18, 2014, http://sugarscience.ucsf.edu/the-growing -concern-of-overconsumption/.

66   *Studies have shown that green . . .:* Paul Grant, "Spearmint Herbal Tea Has Significant Anti-androgen Effects in Polycystic Ovarian Syndrome: A Randomized Controlled Trial," *Phytotherapy Research,* February 2010, doi:10.1002/ptr.2900.

66   *Studies have shown it works . . .:* C. S. Johnston, C. M. Kim, and A. J. Buller, "Vinegar Improves Insulin Sensitivity to a High-Carbohydrate Meal in Subjects with Insulin Resistance or Type 2 Diabetes," *Diabetes Care* 27/1 (January 2004): 281–82, doi:10.2337/diacare.27.1.281.

66   *A sprinkle of ground cinnamon . . .:* Arjuna B. Medagama, "The Glycaemic Outcomes of Cinnamon: A Review of the Experimental Evidence and Clinical Trials," *Nutrition Journal* 14/1 (October 16, 2015), doi:10.1186 /s12937-015-0098-9.

66   *A dash of cayenne pepper . . .:* Shiqi Zhang et al., "Capsaicin Reduces Blood Glucose by Increasing Insulin Levels and Glycogen Content Better Than Capsiate in Streptozotocin-Induced Diabetic Rats," *Journal of Agricultural and Food Chemistry* 65/11 (March 10, 2017): 2323–330, doi:10.1021/acs.jafc.7b00132.

67   *"By providing a sweet taste without any calories . . .":* Sarah Bleich et al., "Artificial Sweeteners," *The Nutrition Source,* January 29, 2016, https:// www.hsph.harvard.edu/nutritionsource/healthy-drinks/artificial-sweeteners/.

67   *A recent study shows that people who drink . . .:* J. A. Nettleton et al., "Diet Soda Intake and Risk of Incident Metabolic Syndrome and Type 2 Diabetes in the Multi-Ethnic Study of Atherosclerosis (MESA)," *Diabetes Care* 32/4 (January 16, 2009): 688–94, doi:10.2337/dc08-1799.

67   *People who consume two or more diet sodas . . .:* Sharon P. G. Fowler, Ken Williams, and Helen P. Hazuda, "Diet Soda Intake Is Associated with Long-Term Increases in Waist Circumference in a Biethnic Cohort of Older Adults: The San Antonio Longitudinal Study of Aging," *Journal of the American Geriatrics Society* 63/4 (March 17, 2015): 708–15, doi:10.1111/jgs.13376.

67   *Studies show that people who consume . . .:* "Hold the Diet Soda? Sweetened Drinks Linked to Depression, Coffee Tied to Lower Risk," *American Academy of Neurology,* January 8, 2013, https://www.aan.com/PressRoom/home/Press Release/1128.

68   *"Women who drink cola daily . . ."*: "Study: Cola Linked to Lower Bone Density in Women," *Tufts University E-News*, October 20, 2006, http://enews.tufts.edu/stories/22/2006/10/20/StudyColaLinkedToLowerBoneDensityInWomen.

69   *"help moderate the hormone imbalance . . ."*: Beata Banaszewska et al., "Effects of Resveratrol on Polycystic Ovary Syndrome: A Double-blind, Randomized, Placebo-controlled Trial," *The Journal of Clinical Endocrinology & Metabolism* 101/11 (October 18, 2016): 4322–328, doi:10.1210/jc.2016-1858.

69   *Black, green:* Shin Nishiumi et al., "Green and Black Tea Suppress Hyperglycemia and Insulin Resistance by Retaining the Expression of Glucose Transporter 4 in Muscle of High-Fat Diet-Fed C57BL/6J Mice," *Journal of Agricultural and Food Chemistry* 58/24 (November 24, 2010): 12916–2923, doi:10.1021/jf102840w; K. Liu et al., "Effect of Green Tea on Glucose Control and Insulin Sensitivity: A Meta-Analysis of 17 Randomized Controlled Trials," *American Journal of Clinical Nutrition* 98/2 (June 26, 2013): 340–48, doi:10.3945/ajcn.112.052746.

69   *ginger:* Natalia De Las Heras et al., "Molecular Factors Involved in the Hypolipidemic- and Insulin-Sensitizing Effects of a Ginger (*Zingiber officinale* Roscoe) Extract in Rats Fed a High-Fat Diet," *Applied Physiology, Nutrition, and Metabolism* 42/2 (November 2, 2016): 209–15, doi:10.1139/apnm-2016-0374.

69   *turmeric:* Roya Navekar et al., "Turmeric Supplementation Improves Serum Glucose Indices and Leptin Levels in Patients with Nonalcoholic Fatty Liver Diseases," *Journal of the American College of Nutrition* 36/4 (May–June, 2017): 261–67, doi:10.1080/07315724.2016.1267597.

69   *Spearmint, red reishi, licorice . . .:* Paul Grant and Shamin Ramasamy, "An Update on Plant Derived Anti-Androgens," *International Journal of Endocrinology and Metabolism* 10/2 (2012): 497–502, doi:10.5812/ijem.3644.

69   *Tea contains an amino acid called L-theanine . . .:* A. C. Nobre, A. Rao, and G. N. Owen, "L-theanine, a Natural Constituent in Tea, and Its Effect on Mental State," *Asia Pacific Journal of Clinical Nutrition* 17/S1 (2008): 168, https://www.ncbi.nlm.nih.gov/pubmed/18296328.

69   *In addition, researchers have found . . .:* Catharine Paddock, "Does a Cup of Tea Reduce Stress?" *Medical News Today*, August 14, 2009, https://www.medicalnewstoday.com/articles/160668.php.

69   *Tea has been used for centuries . . .:* D. Heber et al., "Green Tea, Black Tea, and Oolong Tea Polyphenols Reduce Visceral Fat and Inflammation in Mice Fed High-Fat, High-Sucrose Obesogenic Diets," *Journal of Nutrition* 144/9 (September 2014): 1385–93, doi:10.3945/jn.114.191007.

70   *Studies specifically find that zinc . . .:* Ellen Grant, "Polycystic Ovarian Syndrome: The Metabolic Syndrome Comes to Gynaecology," *The BMJ* 317/7154 (August 1, 1998): 329–32, doi:10.1136/bmj.317.7154.329.

70   *A lack of folate may also result . . .:* M. Ramos et al., "Low Folate Status Is Associated with Impaired Cognitive Function and Dementia in the Sacramento

Area Latino Study on Aging," *American Journal of Clinical Nutrition* 82/6, 1346–52, https://www.ncbi.nlm.nih.gov/pubmed/16332669.

71   *High levels of homocysteine . . . depression:* S. Gilbody, S. Lewis, and T. Lightfoot, "Methylenetetrahydrofolate Reductase (MTHFR) Genetic Polymorphisms and Psychiatric Disorders: A HuGE Review," *American Journal of Epidemiology* 165/1 (October 30, 2006): 1–13, doi:10.1093/aje/kwj347.

71   *High levels of homocysteine . . . migraines:* J. Azimova et al., "Effects of MTHFR Gene Polymorphism on the Clinical and Electrophysiological Characteristics of Migraine," *BMC Neurology* 13/103 (August 5, 2013), doi:10.1186/1471-2377-13-103.

71   *Even when D6D functions normally . . . :* Aliza H. Stark, Michael A. Crawford, and Ram Reifen, "Update on Alpha-Linolenic Acid," *Nutrition Reviews* 66/6 (June 1, 2008): 326–32, doi:10.1111/j.1753-4887.2008.00040.x.

71   *Found in meat, myo-inositol is critical . . . :* Sriramoju M. Kumar et al., "Molecular Level Interaction of the Human Acidic Fibroblast Growth Factor with the Antiangiogenic Agent Inositol Hexaphosphate," *Biochemistry* 49/50 (December 21, 2010): 10756–64, doi:10.1021/bi101318m; Christiaan B. Brink et al., "Effects of Myo-inositol Versus Fluoxetine and Imipramine Pretreatments on Serotonin 5HT2A and Muscarinic Acetylcholine Receptors in Human Neuroblastoma Cells," *Metabolic Brain Disease* 19/1–2 (June 2004): 51–70, doi:10.1023/b:mebr.0000027417.74156.5f.

72   *inducing menses:* E. Papaleo et al., "Myo-inositol in Patients with Polycystic Ovary Syndrome: A Novel Method for Ovulation Induction," *Gynecological Endocrinology* 23/12 (October 10, 2007): 700–703, doi:10.1080/09513590701672405.

72   *reducing acne and hirsutism:* Martino M Zacchè et al., "Efficacy of Myo-inositol in the Treatment of Cutaneous Disorders in Young Women with Polycystic Ovary Syndrome," *Gynecological Endocrinology* 25/8 (August 2009): 508–13, doi:10.1080/09513590903015544.

72   *Studies suggest that women with PCOS . . . :* Nicolas Galazis, Myria Galazi, and William Atiomo, "D-chiro-inositol and Its Significance in Polycystic Ovary Syndrome: A Systematic Review," *Gynecological Endocrinology* 27/4 (December 10, 2010): 256–62, doi:10.3109/09513590.2010.538099.

72   *Low levels of DCI have commonly . . . :* Deepika Garg and Reshef Tal, "Inositol Treatment and ART Outcomes in Women with PCOS," *International Journal of Endocrinology* (October 4, 2016): 1–9, doi:10.1155/2016/1979654.

72   *DCI increases the action of insulin . . . :* John E. Nestler et al., "Ovulatory and Metabolic Effects of D-chiro-inositol in the Polycystic Ovary Syndrome," *Obstetrical & Gynecological Survey* 54/9 (April 29, 1999): 573–74, doi:10.1097/00006254-199909000-00018.

72   *decrease testosterone . . . :* Maria J. Iuorno et al., "Effects of D-chiro-inositol in Lean Women with the Polycystic Ovary Syndrome," *Endocrine Practice* 8/6 (November–December 2002): 417–23, doi:10.4158/ep.8.6.417.

72   *improve IVF outcomes:* S. Colazingari et al., "The Combined Therapy Myo-inositol plus D-chiro-inositol, Rather Than D-chiro-inositol, Is

Able to Improve IVF Outcomes: Results from a Randomized Controlled Trial," *Archives of Gynecology and Obstetrics* 288/6 (December 2013): 1405–11, doi:10.1007/s00404-013-2855-3, https://www.ncbi.nlm.nih.gov/pubmed /23708322.

72   *Three out of four women with PCOS have . . .*: E. Wehr et al., "Association of Hypovitaminosis D with Metabolic Disturbances in Polycystic Ovary Syndrome," *European Journal of Endocrinology* 161/4 (October 1, 2009): 575–82, doi:10.1530/eje-09-0432.

72   *This may exacerbate the symptoms . . .*: Meng-Hsing Wu and Ming-Wei Lin, "The Role of Vitamin D in Polycystic Ovary Syndrome," *Indian Journal of Medical Research* 142/3 (September 2015): 238, doi:10.4103/0971-5916.166527.

72   *increase the risk for multiple sclerosis, inflammation . . .*: "Vitamin D Fact Sheet for Health Professionals," NIH Office of Dietary Supplements, February 11, 2016, https://ods.od.nih.gov/factsheets/VitaminD-HealthProfessional/; Katherine Zeratsky, "Mayo Clinic Q and A: How Much Vitamin D Do I Need?" *Mayo Clinic,* June 5, 2015, https://newsnetwork.mayoclinic.org /discussion/mayo-clinic-q-and-a-how-much-vitamin-d-do-i-need/.

72   *A vitamin-D deficiency may be caused . . .*: Touraj Mahmoudi, "Genetic Variation in the Vitamin D Receptor and Polycystic Ovary Syndrome Risk," *Fertility and Sterility* 92/4 (October 2009): 1381–83, doi:10.1016/j.fertnstert .2009.05.002.

72   *Vitamin D works . . .*: Y. Zhang et al., "Vitamin D Inhibits Monocyte/ Macrophage Proinflammatory Cytokine Production by Targeting MAPK Phosphatase-1," *Journal of Immunology* 188/5 (March 1, 2012): 2127–35, doi:10.4049/jimmunol.1102412.

72   *Moreover, they discovered improvement . . .*: "Researchers Discover How Vitamin D Inhibits Inflammation," *National Jewish Health,* February 23, 2012, https://www.nationaljewish.org/about/news/press-releases/2012/vitd -mechanism.

73   *Studies show that women who use . . .*: M. Palmery et al., "Oral Contraceptives and Changes in Nutritional Requirements," *European Review for Medical and Pharmacological Sciences* 17/13 (July 2013): 1804–13, https:// www.ncbi.nlm.nih.gov/pubmed/23852908; Federico Lussana et al., "Blood Levels of Homocysteine, Folate, Vitamin B_6 and B_{12} in Women Using Oral Contraceptives Compared to Non-users," *Thrombosis Research* 112/1–2 (2003): 37–41, doi:10.1016/j.thromres.2003.11.007; Jennifer McArthur et al., "Biological Variability and Impact of Oral Contraceptives on Vitamins B_6, B_{12} and Folate Status in Women of Reproductive Age," *Nutrients* 5/9 (September 16, 2013): 3634–45, doi:10.3390/nu5093634.

73   *In fact, low levels of B_6 . . .*: Federico Lussana et al., "Blood Levels of Homocysteine, Folate, Vitamin B_6 and B_{12} in Women Using Oral Contraceptives Compared to Non-users," *Thrombosis Research* 112/1–2 (2003): 37–41, doi:10.1016/j.thromres.2003.11.007.

73   *Other studies indicate that the pill . . .*: M. Palmery, A. Saraceno, A. Vaiarelli, and G. Carlomagno, "Oral Contraceptives and Changes in

Nutritional Requirements," *European Review for Medical Pharmacological Sciences* 17/13 (July 2013): 1804–813, https://www.ncbi.nlm.nih.gov/pubmed /23852908.

73 *Meant to lower insulin levels . . . :* David S. H. Bell, "Metformin-Induced Vitamin B_{12} Deficiency Presenting as a Peripheral Neuropathy," *Southern Medical Journal* 103/3 (May 3, 2010): 265–67, doi:10.1097/smj .0b013e3181ce0e4d.

75 *Women with PCOS are nineteen times . . . :* Faranak Sharifi et al., "Serum Magnesium Concentrations in Polycystic Ovary Syndrome and Its Association with Insulin Resistance," *Gynecological Endocrinology* 28/1 (June 23, 2011): 7–11, doi:10.3109/09513590.2011.579663.

78 *People who regularly eat dark chocolate . . . :* Beatrice A. Golomb, "Association Between More Frequent Chocolate Consumption and Lower Body Mass Index," *Archives of Internal Medicine* 172/6 (March 26, 2012): 519, doi:10.1001/archinternmed.2011.2100.

78 *Studies indicate that regularly eating . . . :* D. Mastroiacovo et al., "Cocoa Flavanol Consumption Improves Cognitive Function, Blood Pressure Control, and Metabolic Profile in Elderly Subjects: The Cocoa, Cognition, and Aging (CoCoA) Study—A Randomized Controlled Trial," *American Journal of Clinical Nutrition* 101/3 (December 17, 2014): 538–48, doi:10.3945/ajcn.114.092189.

78 *Studies show that dark chocolate reduces . . . :* Francois-Pierre J. Martin et al., "Metabolic Effects of Dark Chocolate Consumption on Energy, Gut Microbiota, and Stress-Related Metabolism in Free-Living Subjects," *Journal of Proteome Research* 8/12 (December 2009): 5568–79, doi:10.1021/pr900607v.

78 *A study published in the* American Journal of Clinical Nutrition *. . . :* Davide Grassi et al., "Short-Term Administration of Dark Chocolate Is Followed by a Significant Increase in Insulin Sensitivity and a Decrease in Blood Pressure in Healthy Persons," *American Journal of Clinical Nutrition* 81/3 (March 2005): 611–14, http://ajcn.nutrition.org/content/81/3/611.abstract.

78 *In a nine-year Japanese study . . . :* Jia-Yi Dong et al., "Chocolate Consumption and Risk of Stroke Among Men And Women: A Large Population-Based, Prospective Cohort Study," *Atherosclerosis* 260 (May 2017): 8–12, doi:10.1016/j.atherosclerosis.2017.03.004.

Chapter 5. Move like a PCOS Diva

85 *Studies indicate that 25 percent of women . . . :* Bulent O. Yildiz et al., "Stability of Adrenocortical Steroidogenesis over Time in Healthy Women and Women with Polycystic Ovary Syndrome," *Journal of Clinical Endocrinology & Metabolism* 89/11 (November 1, 2004): 5558–62, doi:10.1210/jc.2004-0934.

87 *HIIT also significantly lowers insulin . . . :* Stephen H. Boutcher, "High-Intensity Intermittent Exercise and Fat Loss," *Journal of Obesity* 2011 (November 24, 2010): 1–10, doi:10.1155/2011/868305.

89 *Studies galore demonstrate its benefits . . . :* Ram Nidhi et al., "Effect of a Yoga Program on Glucose Metabolism and Blood Lipid Levels in Adolescent

Girls with Polycystic Ovary Syndrome," *International Journal of Gynecology & Obstetrics* 118/1 (April 14, 2012): 37–41, doi:10.1016/j.ijgo.2012.01.027.

91   *Lack of sleep can wreak serious havoc . . .:* "Sleep and Disease Risk," *Healthy Sleep*, Harvard Medical School, December 18, 2007, http://healthy sleep.med.harvard.edu/healthy/matters/consequences/sleep-and-disease-risk.

92   *Women with PCOS are at least thirty times…:* Esra Tasali, Eve Van Cauter, and David A. Ehrmann, "Relationships Between Sleep Disordered Breathing and Glucose Metabolism in Polycystic Ovary Syndrome," *Journal of Clinical Endocrinology & Metabolism* 91/1 (January 1, 2006): 36–42, doi:10.1210/jc.2005 -1084.

Chapter 6. Prepare for Success

101   *They have also been linked . . .:* João Ricardo Araújo, Fátima Martel, and Elisa Keating, "Exposure to Non-nutritive Sweeteners During Pregnancy and Lactation: Impact in Programming of Metabolic Diseases in the Progeny Later in Life," *Reproductive Toxicology* 49 (November 2014): 196–201, doi:10.1016/j.reprotox.2014.09.007.

102   *They are a weak estrogenic . . .:* Edwin J. Routledge et al., "Some Alkyl Hydroxy Benzoate Preservatives (Parabens) Are Estrogenic," *Toxicology and Applied Pharmacology* 153/1 (November 1998): 12–19, doi:10.1006/taap.1998 .8544.

102   *have been shown to affect sleep . . .:* John D. Stokes and Charles L. Scudder, "The Effect of Butylated Hydroxyanisole and Butylated Hydroxytoluene on Behavioral Development of Mice," *Developmental Psychobiology* 7/4 (July 1974): 343–50, doi:10.1002/dev.420070411.

102   *metabolism and nutrition disorders:* "Sodium Benzoate/Sodium Phenylacetate Side Effects in Detail," *Drugs.com*, accessed October 26, 2017, https://www.drugs.com/sfx/sodium-benzoate-sodium-phenylacetate-side -effects.html.

102   *liver and kidney damage:* R. S. Lanigan and T. A. Yamarik, "Final Report on the Safety Assessment of BHT," *International Journal of Toxicology* 21/2 suppl (2002): 19–94, doi:10.1080/10915810290096513.

102   *and cancer:* "14th Report on Carcinogens," *National Institute of Environmental Health Sciences*, November 3, 2016, https://ntp.niehs.nih.gov /pubhealth/roc/index-1.html.

102   *It has been banned in one hundred countries . . .:* Brett Israel, "Brominated Battle: Soda Chemical Has Cloudy Health History," *Scientific American*, December 12, 2011, https://www.scientificamerican.com/article/soda-chemical -cloudy-health-history/.

102   *more likely to develop diabetes . . .:* Renata Micha, Sarah K. Wallace, and Dariush Mozaffarian, "Red and Processed Meat Consumption and Risk of Incident Coronary Heart Disease, Stroke, and Diabetes: A Systematic Review and Meta-Analysis," *Circulation* 121/21 (June 1, 2010): 2271–83, doi:10.1161 /CIRCULATIONAHA.109.924977; Katherine Zeratsky, "The Unhealthy

Preservative Hiding in Processed Meats," *Mayo Clinic*, April 10, 2015, http://www.mayoclinic.org/healthy-lifestyle/nutrition-and-healthy-eating/expert-answers/sodium-nitrate/faq-20057848.

102   *to form nitrosamine, a highly carcinogenic substance:* "IARC Monographs Evaluate Consumption of Red Meat and Processed Meat," *International Agency for Research on Cancer*, World Health Organization, October 26, 2015, https://www.iarc.fr/en/media-centre/pr/2015/pdfs/pr240_E.pdf.

102   *Artificial flavors and colors are linked to . . . :* Christopher Gavigan, "Food Dyes: Red Does Not Mean GO," *Huffington Post*, September 23, 2013, http://www.huffingtonpost.com/christopher-gavigan/food-dye_b_3792860.html.

102   *In addition, they can contain . . . :* "CFR–Code of Federal Regulations Title 21," *US Food & Drug Administration*, April 1, 2016, http://www.accessdata.fda.gov/scripts/cdrh/cfdocs/cfcfr/CFRSearch.cfm?CFRPart=73&showFR=1.

114   *"If you have an impulse to act . . .":* Mel Robbins, "The 5 Second Rule," April 2, 2016, http://melrobbins.com/the-5-second-rule/.

116   *A sprinkle of cayenne will wake . . . :* K. Chaiyasit, W. Khovidhunkit, and S. Wittayalertpanya, "Pharmacokinetic and the Effect of Capsaicin in Capsicum frutescens on Decreasing Plasma Glucose Level," *Journal of the Medical Association of Thailand* 92/1 (January 2009): 108–13, https://www.ncbi.nlm.nih.gov/pubmed/19260251.

116   *Studies have shown that it increases . . . :* Masayuki Saito and Takeshi Yoneshiro, "Capsinoids and Related Food Ingredients Activating Brown Fat Thermogenesis and Reducing Body Fat in Humans," *Current Opinion in Lipidology* 24/1 (February 2013): 71–77, doi:10.1097/mol.0b013e32835a4f40; Stephen Whiting, Emma Derbyshire, and B. K. Tiwari, "Capsaicinoids and Capsinoids. A Potential Role for Weight Management? A Systematic Review of the Evidence," *Appetite* 59/2 (2012): 341–48, doi:10.1016/j.appet.2012.05.015.

117   *Ginger has anti-inflammatory compounds . . . :* Sepide Mahluji et al., "Effects of Ginger (*Zingiber officinale*) on Plasma Glucose Level, HbA1c and Insulin Sensitivity in Type 2 Diabetic Patients," *International Journal of Food Sciences and Nutrition* 64/6 (September 2013): 682–86, doi:10.3109/09637486.2013.775223; Yiming Li et al., "Preventive and Protective Properties of Zingiber officinale (Ginger) in Diabetes Mellitus, Diabetic Complications, and Associated Lipid and Other Metabolic Disorders: A Brief Review," *Evidence-Based Complementary and Alternative Medicine* 2012 (2012): 1–10, doi:10.1155/2012/516870.

117   *A teaspoon or two of apple cider vinegar . . . :* C. S. Johnston, C. M. Kim, and A. J. Buller, "Vinegar Improves Insulin Sensitivity to a High-Carbohydrate Meal in Subjects with Insulin Resistance or Type 2 Diabetes," *Diabetes Care* 27/1 (January 2004): 281–82, doi:10.2337/diacare.27.1.281.

117   *Numerous studies have shown . . . :* Ahmed Sahib, "Antidiabetic and Antioxidant Effect of Cinnamon in Poorly Controlled Type-2 Diabetic Iraqi Patients: A Randomized, Placebo-Controlled Clinical Trial," *Journal of Intercultural Ethnopharmacology* 5/2 (2016): 108, doi:10.5455/jice.20160217044511.

117   *Curcumin, the active ingredient . . . :* Nita Chainani-Wu, "Safety and Anti-Inflammatory Activity of Curcumin: A Component of Tumeric (Curcuma longa)," *Journal of Alternative and Complementary Medicine* 9/1 (February 2003): 161–68, doi:10.1089/107555303321223035.

117   *it can help with diabetes:* Omotayo O. Erejuwa, Siti A. Sulaiman, and Mohd S. Ab Wahab, "Honey—A Novel Antidiabetic Agent," *International Journal of Biological Sciences* 8/6 (July 7, 2012): 913–34, doi:10.7150/ijbs.3697.

117   *sleep problems:* Ron Fessenden, "The Honey Revolution," *Living Honey*, accessed October 26, 2017, http://www.livinghoney.biz/the-honey-revolution .html.

117   *coughs:* Olabisi Oduwole et al., "Honey for Acute Cough in Children," *Evidence-Based Child Health: A Cochrane Review Journal* 9/2 (March 14, 2014): 401–44, doi:10.1002/ebch.1970.

117   *wound healing:* P. Lusby, A. Coombes, and J. M. Wilkinson, "Honey: A Potent Agent for Wound Healing?" *Journal of Wound, Ostomy, and Continence Nursing* 29/6 (November 2002): 295–300, doi:10.1067/mjw.2002.129073.

122   *This will increase your energy . . . :* A. Franke et al., "Postprandial Walking but Not Consumption of Alcoholic Digestifs or Espresso Accelerates Gastric Emptying in Healthy Volunteers," *Journal of Gastrointestinal and Liver Diseases* 17/1 (March 2008): 27–31, https://www.ncbi.nlm.nih.gov/pubmed /18392240; Sheri R. Colberg et al., "Postprandial Walking Is Better for Lowering the Glycemic Effect of Dinner Than Pre-Dinner Exercise in Type 2 Diabetic Individuals," *Journal of the American Medical Directors Association* 10/6 (July 2009): 394–97, doi:10.1016/j.jamda.2009.03.015; L. Dipietro et al., "Three 15-Min Bouts of Moderate Postmeal Walking Significantly Improves 24-h Glycemic Control in Older People at Risk for Impaired Glucose Tolerance," *Diabetes Care* 36/10 (October 2013): 3262–68, doi:10.2337 /dc13–0084.

123   *In addition, tablet readers reported . . . :* Anne-Marie Chang et al., "Evening Use of Light-Emitting eReaders Negatively Affects Sleep, Circadian Timing, and Next-Morning Alertness," *PNAS*, December 22, 2014, doi:10.1073/pnas.1418490112.

125   *Without adequate magnesium . . . :* Tommi Möykkynen et al., "Magnesium Potentiation of the Function of Native and Recombinant GABA(A) Receptors," *Neuroreport* 12/10 (July 2001): 2175–79, doi:10.1097/00001756 -200107200-00026.

125   *Magnesium can also help reduce . . . :* S. W. Golf et al., "Plasma Aldosterone, Cortisol and Electrolyte Concentrations in Physical Exercise After Magnesium Supplementation," *Journal of Clinical Chemistry and Clinical Biochemistry* 22/11 (November 1984): 717–21, doi:10.1515/cclm.1984.22.11.717.

126   *Lavender is one . . . :* Peir Hossein Koulivand, Maryam Khaleghi Ghadiri, and Ali Gorji, "Lavender and the Nervous System," *Evidence-Based Complementary and Alternative Medicine*, March 14, 2013, doi:10.1155/2013 /681304.

126   *Bergamot, known for its ability . . .:* Michelle Navarra et al., *"Citrus Bergamia* Essential Oil: From Basic Research to Clinical Application," *Frontiers in Pharmacology,* March 2, 2015, doi:10.3389/fphar.2015.00036.

126   *Ylang-ylang activates . . .:* Tapanee Hongratanaworakit and Gerhard Buchbauer. "Relaxing Effect of Ylang Oil on Humans After Transdermal Absorption," *Phytotherapy Research* 20/9 (September 20, 2006): 758–63, doi:10.1002/ptr.1950.

126   *Clary sage is one . . .:* Kyung-Bok Lee, Eun Cho, and Young-Sook Kang, "Changes in 5-Hydroxytryptamine and Cortisol Plasma Levels in Menopausal Women After Inhalation of Clary Sage Oil," *Phytotherapy Research* 28/12 (November 2014): 1897, doi:10.1002/ptr.5268.

127   *Researchers at the University of Surrey . . .:* "Reading 'Can Help Reduce Stress,'" *The Telegraph,* March 30, 2009, http://www.telegraph.co.uk/news /health/news/5070874/Reading-can-help-reduce-stress.html.

128   *It has been shown that you may need . . .:* Anantha Lakkakula et al., "Repeated Taste Exposure Increases Liking for Vegetables by Low-Income Elementary School Children," *Appetite* 55/2 (October 2010): 226–31, doi:10.1016/j.appet.2010.06.003.

Chapter 8. Week Two: Live

171   *creative, insightful, inspiring . . .: INFJ type, Sixteen Personalities test,* https://www.16personalities.com/infj-strengths-and-weaknesses.

178   *A double-blind study . . .:* Andrew Steptoe et al., "The Effects of Tea on a Psychophysiological Stress Responsivity and Post-Stress Recovery: A Randomised Double-Blind Trial," *Psychopharmacology* 190/1 (January 30, 2006): 81–89, doi:10.1007/s00213-006-0573-2.

180   *I soon was surprised to learn . . .:* Jessie X. Fan et al., "Moderate to Vigorous Physical Activity and Weight Outcomes: Does Every Minute Count?" *American Journal of Health Promotion* 28/1 (September–October 2013): 41–49, doi:10.4278/ajhp.120606-qual-286.

188   *Dr. Aron has identified people . . .:* David McNamee, "'Sensitive People' Show Heightened Activity in Empathy-Related Brain Regions," *Medical News Today,* June 23, 2014, http://www.medicalnewstoday.com/articles/278589.php.

Chapter 9. Week Three: Thrive

192   *Most alarming for women with PCOS . . .:* "Chronic Stress Puts Your Health at Risk," *Mayo Clinic,* April 21, 2016, http://www.mayoclinic.org /healthy-lifestyle/stress-management/in-depth/stress/art-20046037.

192   *It may also ease symptoms of anxiety, depression . . .:* "Meditation: In Depth," *National Center for Complementary and Integrative Health,* September 07, 2017, https://nccih.nih.gov/health/meditation/overview.htm.

207   *Research shows that clutter may . . .:* Lenny R. Vartanian, Brian Wansink, and Kristin M. Kernan, "Clutter, Chaos, and Overconsumption," *Environment and Behavior* 29/2 (February 2, 2016), doi:10.1177/0013916516628178.

207   *Clutter caused people to lose focus . . .:* S. McMains and S. Kastner, "Interactions of Top-Down and Bottom-Up Mechanisms in Human Visual Cortex," *Journal of Neuroscience* 31/2 (January 12, 2011): 587–97, doi:10.1523/JNEUROSCI.3766–10.2011.

208   *Dr. Joel Pearson, a brain scientist . . .:* Dana Dovey, "The Therapeutic Science of Adult Coloring Books: How This Childhood Pastime Helps Adults Relieve Stress," *Medical Daily*, September 06, 2016, http://www.medicaldaily.com/therapeutic-science-adult-coloring-books-how-childhood-pastime-helps-adults-356280.

209   *A 2005 study concurred, demonstrating . . .:* Nancy A. Curry and Tim Kasser, "Can Coloring Mandalas Reduce Anxiety?" *Art Therapy* 22/2 (2005): 81–85, doi:10.1080/07421656.2005.10129441.

209   *Studies have shown that art therapy . . .:* Heather L. Stuckey and Jeremy Nobel, "The Connection Between Art, Healing, and Public Health: A Review of Current Literature," *American Journal of Public Health* 100/2 (February 2010): 254–63, doi:10.2105/ajph.2008.15649.

210   *This type of meditation has been shown . . .:* Barbara L. Fredrickson et al., "Open Hearts Build Lives: Positive Emotions, Induced Through Loving-Kindness Meditation, Build Consequential Personal Resources," *Journal of Personality and Social Psychology* 95/5 (November 2008): 1045–62, doi:10.1037/a0013262.

210   *helps reduce self-criticism:* Ben Shahar et al., "A Wait-List Randomized Controlled Trial of Loving-Kindness Meditation Programme for Self-Criticism," *Clinical Psychology & Psychotherapy* 22/4 (July 16, 2014): 346–56, doi:10.1002/cpp.1893.

214   *Research at Harvard Medical School . . .:* Kathleen K. S. Hui et al., "Acupuncture Modulates the Limbic System and Subcortical Gray Structures of the Human Brain: Evidence from fMRI Studies in Normal Subjects," *Human Brain Mapping* 9/1 (2000): 13–25, doi:10.1002/(sici)1097-0193(2000)9:1<13::aid-hbm2>3.0.co;2-f.

Chapter 10. Moving Forward

218   *In fact, an unhealthy microbiome . . .:* Jim Parker, "Emerging Concepts in the Pathogenesis and Treatment of Polycystic Ovary Syndrome," *Current Women's Health Reviews* 10/2 (2015): 107–12, doi:10.2174/1573404811666150214004706.

218   *Studies indicate that broad-spectrum antibiotics . . .:* Anthony Samsel and Stephanie Seneff, "Glyphosate's Suppression of Cytochrome P450 Enzymes and Amino Acid Biosynthesis by the Gut Microbiome: Pathways to Modern Diseases," *Entropy* 15/4 (April 18, 2013): 1416–63, doi:10.3390/e15041416.

218   *Not only is it possible to heal . . .:* Kristin Sohn and Mark A. Underwood, "Prenatal and Postnatal Administration of Prebiotics and Probiotics," *Seminars in Fetal and Neonatal Medicine* 22/5 (September 2017): 284–89, doi:10.1016/j.siny.2017.07.002; R. Cabrera-Rubio et al., "The Human Milk Microbiome Changes over Lactation and Is Shaped by Maternal Weight and Mode of Delivery," *American Journal of Clinical Nutrition* 96/3 (September 25, 2012): 544–51, doi:10.3945/ajcn.112.037382.

219   *Your body's natural estrogen . . .:* E. Diamanti-Kandarakis, J. P. Bourguignon, and L. C. Giudice, "Endocrine-Disrupting Chemicals: An Endocrine Society Scientific Statement," *Endocrinology Review* (June 30, 2009): 293–342, doi:10.1210/er.2009–0002.

221   *Several studies have hinted . . .:* M. Hudecova et al., "Long-term Follow-up of Patients with Polycystic Ovary Syndrome: Reproductive Outcome and Ovarian Reserve," *Human Reproduction* 24/5 (May 2009): 1176–83, doi:10.1093/humrep/den482; F. Tehrani et al., "Is Polycystic Ovary Syndrome an Exception for Reproductive Aging?" *Human Reproduction* 25/7 (2010): 1775–81, doi:10.1093/humrep/deq088.

222   *They found that the beta-endorphin serum level . . .:* Marta Kialka et al., "Pressure Pain Threshold and β-Endorphins Plasma Level Are Higher in Lean Polycystic Ovary Syndrome Women," *Endocrine Abstracts,* September 7, 2016, doi:10.1530/endoabs.41.ep751.

222   *It explains that women with this disorder . . .:* Ricardo Azziz, Daniel A. Dumesic, and Mark Goodzari, "Polycystic Ovary Syndrome: An Ancient Disorder?" *Fertility and Sterility* 95/5 (April 2011): 1544–48, doi:10.1016/j .fertnstert.2010.09.032.

222   *According to a 2000 analysis . . .:* J. V. Zborowski et al., "Bone Mineral Density, Androgens, and the Polycystic Ovary: The Complex and Controversial Issue of Androgenic Influence in Female Bone," *Journal of Clinical Endocrinology and Metabolism* 85/10 (October 1, 2000), 3496–3506.

222   *Their higher testosterone levels . . .:* André Aleman et al., "A Single Administration of Testosterone Improves Visuospatial Ability in Young Women," *Psychoneuroendocrinology* 29/5 (June 2004): 612–17, doi:10.1016 /s0306-4530(03)00089-1; J. A. Barry, H. S. K. Parekh, and P. J. Hardiman, "Visual-Spatial Cognition in Women with Polycystic Ovarian Syndrome: The Role of Androgens," *Human Reproduction* 28/10 (August 14, 2013): 2832–37, doi:10.1093/humrep/det335.

222   *A 2014 study examined . . .:* Gislaine Satyko Kogure et al., "Women with Polycystic Ovary Syndrome Have Greater Muscle Strength Irrespective of Body Composition," *Gynecological Endocrinology* 31/3 (October 28, 2014): 237–42, doi:10.3109/09513590.2014.982083.

222   *Research suggests that feedback . . .:* Pranjal H. Mehta et al., "Hormonal Underpinnings of Status Conflict: Testosterone and Cortisol Are Related to Decisions and Satisfaction in the Hawk-Dove Game," *Hormones and Behavior* 92 (June 2017): 141–54, doi:10.1016/j.yhbeh.2017.03.009.

222   *When asked whether they would take a job . . .*: P. Sapienza, L. Zingales, and D. Maestripieri, "Gender Differences in Financial Risk Aversion and Career Choices Are Affected by Testosterone," *Proceedings of the National Academy of Sciences* 106/36 (2009): 15268–73, doi:10.1073/pnas.0907352106.

Chapter 11. Recipes

247   *Research shows that women who have . . .*: M. J. Brown, "Carotenoid Bioavailability Is Higher from Salads Ingested with Full-Fat Than with Fat-Reduced Salad Dressings as Measured with Electrochemical Detection," *American Journal of Clinical Nutrition* (August 2004): 396–403, https://www.ncbi.nlm.nih.gov/pubmed/15277161.

Index